EAT RIGHT

Learn how a good diet can help you
stay healthy and live longer

Jairo A. Puentes MD

Copyright © 2024 by Jairo A. Puentes MD.

ISBN: 979-8-89465-092-0 (sc)
ISBN: 979-8-89465-093-7 (e)

All rights reserved. No part of this publication may be reproduced, distributed, or transmitted in any form or by any means, including photocopying, recording, or other electronic or mechanical methods, without the prior written permission of the author, except in the case of brief quotations embodied in critical reviews and certain other noncommercial uses permitted by copyright law.

Printed in the United States of America.

Integrity Publishing
39343 Harbor Hills Blvd Lady Lake, FL 32159

www.integrity-publishing.com

Dedication

This book is dedicated to my beautiful wife, Clara, an excellent companion and a source of inspiration. I hope our love and happiness can inspire my patients and readers to eat the right foods and live healthier and longer lives.

CONTENTS

Preface vii

Introduction xiii

Chapter 1: The Digestive System. 1

Chapter 2: What is the microbiome? 15

Chapter 3: How Can a Balanced Diet Improve Your Health and Quality of Life? 45

Chapter 4: Vitamins, Probiotics, Prebiotics, Minerals, and Supplements 89

Chapter 5: Longevity and Aging 132

Chapter 6: Appendix A: Healthy Smoothies and Recipes. 155

Appendix B: Resources 164

Bibliography and Selected References 167

Additional books researched 175

Index. 185

PREFACE

Am I eating the right food? Is this food healthy or harmful? Have these thoughts ever crossed your mind? How do you know if what you put in your mouth is good and not damaging your body, making you sick, or leading you to an illness or premature death?

When we are young, we rarely think about such things. We eat junk food because it is sweet or tastes good. But what happens after the food enters our stomach? Most people don't give it much thought.

Food brings us joy, satisfaction, energy, and pleasure. But most people never think about what happens inside the digestive system-how the food is processed and transformed into simple nutrients and elements before entering the bloodstream to make new tissues, provide energy, and build proteins to maintain our body's functions.

As time passes, you may begin to gain weight or feel constantly tired, experience frequent diarrhea, or feel nauseous after eating certain foods. You may hear of a friend or relative who had a heart attack or stroke at a young age. It is shocking to think food had something to do with it. You start to wonder.

We might also hear your sister or mother has diabetes. You wonder why-after all, you eat the same foods at home. Grandma and Grandpa also say that their doctor told them they have nerve or kidney damage. But why, you ask? They don't eat junk food, yet they're sick too. Why?

As you ask these questions, you realize that food might be involved. But how did this illness develop? What's really going on? Is it genetic?

You love your family, and you start to worry. What can you do to help? Am I going to get sick like them, too? You wonder.

To learn more, you go online looking for information. However, you often find different opinions and terminology hard to comprehend. You may feel confused and unsure where to go for reliable and accurate information.

I am a doctor with over fifty years of clinical experience, treating thousands of people. I am also a former professor of medicine who has been reviewing scientific articles and writing to help people find good information among the clutter on the internet and popular magazines.

My wife and I wrote this book to help you answer many questions about the best diets for optimizing body function and to share our personal experiences of staying healthy and youthful.

We are living proof of this prescription. At our age, we enjoy good health and vitality and look healthier than people of similar chronological age. Physically, our bodies appear more youthful than many of our peers.

Biologically, we are 20 to 30 years younger than most of them, thanks to our lifestyle, diet, and carefully chosen supplements.

I invite you to join me through the exciting world of our digestive system to learn what happens to the food we ingest, how it is processed nourish the billions of cells in our body and the trillions of microbes in our microbiome, and how these microbes help us digest food and produce hormones, peptides, and chemicals that help our cells to grow healthy, strengthen our immune system, and create the proteins and chemicals necessary to improve our health and extend our lives.

I will be your guide, explaining where we are during our journey, what is happening, and how nutrients keep our cells alive and functional, ensuring that when we eat right, we can live as many years as possible in good health.

When you finish this book, I hope you apply what you've learned to eat right, enhance your health, prevent damage to your body, and live a longer, healthier life.

Many things have happened since my wife and I wrote the book *Living Longer and Reversing Aging*, published in 2018.

To provide more information available to our readers, patients, and followers, we created a book for each letter of our DRESS-SS prescription: Diet, Rest, Exercise, Sleep, Stress Management, Sexuality, and Spirituality.

To this end, this book is the first of our *Living Longer* series, focused on diets and the digestive system. We continue to search for unbiased and current information out of the clutter of conflicting and sometimes confusing information about diets. We bring you our combined experience, practical knowledge, and more than fifty years of clinical expertise.

The fields of cellular biology, genetics, nutrition, and biochemistry-particularly the study of cellular processes and the chemical pathways involved in forming proteins are advancing substantially. These proteins are responsible for conveying information to different cells to initiate or activate chemical processes. In addition, technological advances in AI and quantum computing are opening new areas of research and understanding how nutrients interact to carry out the functions necessary to make our lives healthier and better.

We explain these advances in this book. We are on the threshold of a revolution that could extend both our health span and lifespan indefinitely. Forward thinkers like Elon Musk are already planning to travel to Mars and populate other planets.

To that end, they must prepare to understand our biological processes to ensure that the future astronauts remain healthy, even with limited resources.

One of the first challenges is maintaining a balanced diet with a healthy microbiome. In the meantime, we are learning why our bodies deteriorate as we age and how to combat these deficiencies and related problems.

Medicine as it is today will change dramatically in the following decades. The emphasis on preventing dysfunctional processes with proper nutrients and the use of supplements to eliminate or reduce senescent cells contributing to chronic inflammation is advancing and promising.

It is gratifying to understand how our immune system not only protects us but can also damage our organs and tissues.

With the development of the COVID-19 vaccine and the pandemic, our scientists understand better how our immune system can be overwhelmed to the point of causing so much damage, the development of autoimmune diseases, and premature organ degeneration.

Applying this knowledge to prevent such malfunctions is a powerful way to extend our longevity and lead healthier lives.

Other outstanding events since the writing of our first book include:

1) The COVID-19 pandemic, which devastated the lives of millions of people globally;
2) The development of artificial intelligence (AI) and quantum computing technology; and
3) Significant advances in longevity and anti-aging medicine.

We believe we are entering a new era of advanced medicine and technology we have never seen before.

Our health and longevity are expected to change significantly in the coming decades. According to some estimates, more than two million centenarians will be alive by 2050.

Scientists are making significant advances in extending the lives of mice and other animals, with potential applications to humans.

New senolytic drugs to remove zombie or senescent cells are extending the life of mice in the laboratory. Metformin and resveratrol chemicals derived from plants that help to prolong life, are some. All these lab experiments and chemicals are helping to extend life and improve health.

It is possible to reach the age of 120 or 130, what's more important is enhancing health and conquering many diseases associated with aging.

Many billionaire investors are now supporting this type of research. Scientists can repair DNA damage by activating the epigenome, which controls the role of proteins and enzymes.

Longevity genes are activated by factors acting on the epigenome.

In this book, I've added a chapter about longevity and aging to explain more deeply how the epigenome can modify the genome to reverse our biological clock and affect the aging process.

I also explain why many of the diseases that affect us as we age are preventable and what you can do to address them.

Reversing and preventing illness is the most intelligent and efficient way to avoid disability and premature death.

I specialized in Physical Medicine and Rehabilitation, treating patients with severe brain, spinal cord, and orthopedic injuries for many years.

Early in my practice, I also developed wellness and cardiac rehabilitation programs for patients with coronary artery disease, both before and after surgical interventions, bypass surgery, or heart transplantation, with outstanding leaders in their fields.

It was then that I realized the need to take action before these problems developed, as they were causing so much pain and suffering.

For many people, in many cases, it was impossible to reverse the damage. Later, I became aware of the importance of eliminating plaque in obstructed coronary arteries through rigorous diets. Dr. Caldwell Esselstyn, in his book *Prevent and Reverse Heart Disease* (2008), made me believe that reversing an illness like coronary heart disease through diet was possible.

I wondered: why not apply the same approach to stroke, Alzheimer's, and all degenerative diseases primarily affecting seniors?

It all made sense. If, by analogy, planes were crashing every day, killing thousands of people, the most logical intervention was to find out why this was happening to prevent more deaths.

Medicine's failure to prevent or reverse such morbidity and mortality was unacceptable. But it was not happening. Giving patients medications, doing more bypasses, or installing stents was not a real solution. Waiting for a plane crash was not acceptable either. The same is true for the medical profession-waiting until people become sick or die of preventable diseases is unacceptable. From that point, I began to inquire and learn how to reverse diseases and identify the common factors leading to these fatal outcomes.

I realized what the problem was. Medical education, doctors, and pharmaceutical companies had divided the body into their areas of interest, neglecting the whole, thus limiting the scope for natural healing and searching for common factors leading to chronic illness responsible for premature aging.

Fortunately, a few doctors and scientists began exploring the genome and the factors that drive genes to express themselves.

Learning to suppress the expression of defective genes or their variants emerged as a way to prevent many chronic illnesses and reverse the damage caused. Advances in nutrition and how nutritional factors trigger or control inflammation have been encouraging.

Every day, we learn more about how chemicals derived from plants can activate pathways to improve longevity and reverse chronic inflammation.

Plants are like medicines; they contain all the nutrients, antioxidants, and chemicals that help us stay healthy or fight disease. We hope this book will enlighten you and guide you to eat the right foods to stay healthy and prevent many illnesses. It will also explain how you can reverse an illness by adjusting your diet without the use of medications.

Jairo A. Puentes MD
Clara I. Puentes

INTRODUCTION

Why Call This Book "Eat Right"?

We consume all kinds of foods without fully understanding how they are processed in our digestive system before being absorbed to feed our cells and organs. Not all foods are good nutrients; some can damage our organs and negatively affect our health. With more knowledge and understanding of the role of micronutrients, we can educate ourselves and our children to choose foods that enhance our health and help prevent many chronic and degenerative diseases.

Writing a nonfiction book requires thorough research, subject knowledge, experience, and the ability to express all this information clearly to the public. My goal is to cut through the clutter and misinformation prevalent today.

I am a doctor with over fifty years of clinical and teaching experience. I could write a book filled with scientific jargon and complexities, but such effort would be limited to doctors or scientists. As an educator, I want to talk directly to you-the public-particularly those who have never gone to college or taken a course in biology or nutrition. I use simple language, relatable examples, and analogies to make complex concepts easier to understand. These associations help for better recall and keep our memory fresh and ready to remember something difficult to follow or understand.

Eating right is vital for our survival. Without proper food or water, we cannot live.

In this book, I will help you to understand why you are gaining weight and why most diets fail to help you lose it. You will also learn why a diet rich in animal foods and saturated fats raises insulin levels, causing insulin resistance and obesity. You will learn how to reverse such problems by switching to a plant-based diet. If you use supplements or diets with whey protein rich in BCAAs (Branch Chain Amino Acids) to increase muscle mass, you are at risk of diabetes and obesity. I will explain how foods rich in these amino acids and methionine can shorten your lifespan and increase your risk of diabetes and weight gain. Most degenerative and cardiovascular diseases are preventable, and I will explain how you can achieve this goal of better health and extended longevity through a plant-based diet.

Several studies demonstrate that Vegans are less likely to gain weight and have a lower risk of heart disease, stroke, Alzheimer's, and degenerative diseases compared to those people whose diet is rich in animal foods. We will review different diets and scientists' findings from the Blue Zones, regions where many centenarians live and still enjoy better health than people living in urban centers worldwide.

Saturated fats in animal food and excessive protein density in animal sources are more detrimental than plant-based food that doesn't contain saturated fats or excessive harmful protein concentrations such as methionine, leucine, and isoleucine.

Chapter One will review the digestive system. It is essential to understand the different roles each segment of the digestive system plays in processing our foods and how they transform into simple elements to be absorbed throughout the intestinal wall. Additionally, this chapter will explain what happens to the remaining food in the intestine as it undergoes a process of elimination.

Chapter Two explains how good bacteria, known as the microbiome, help transform food into amino acids, fats, and nutrients. This chapter also describes how bacteria help the creation of hormones and nutrients that may be unavailable in our diets. The understanding of the microbiome is ongoing and is advancing. All this knowledge has been going on for the past two decades and has become one of the most fascinating research areas. Many autoimmune diseases begin at this level and will explain how a more permeable intestine or "leaky gut" leads to many autoimmune disorders, food sensitivities, and chronic illness.

Chapter Three explains diets in more detail and why they fail.

Chapter Four describes the role of vitamins, minerals, and supplements.

Chapter Five provides information about how to live healthier with the appropriate diet and live longer as we age. This chapter also reviews the state of research conducted to expand our longevity and rejuvenation.

Finally, in Chapters Six, Appendixes A and B, we will provide recipes for delicious and nutritious smoothies and recipes for a healthier diet. Additionally, you'll find information on resources, testing, and laboratories that offer specific tests to evaluate our microbiome and food sensitivities.

CHAPTER 1

The Digestive System

Our digestive system is the port of entry to our foods and nutrients. This organ interacts with all organ systems, particularly the immune and the brain. Without a functioning digestive system, we cannot survive for long or enjoy a healthier life. Reviewing and understanding this vital system, which is the key to survival, is essential to understanding the best foods to eat and which ones to avoid.

What is the digestive system?

Your digestive system is a network of organs that help you digest and absorb nutrition from your food. It includes your gastrointestinal (GI) tract and your biliary system. Your GI tract is a series of hollow organs that are all connected, leading from your mouth to your anus. Your biliary system is a network of three organs that deliver bile and enzymes to your GI tract and bile ducts, aiding digestion.

Anatomy

What Organs Make up the Digestive System?

The main organs that make up your digestive system are the organs known as your gastrointestinal (GI) tract. They are your mouth, esophagus, stomach, small intestine, large intestine, and anus. Supporting your GI organs along the way are your pancreas, gallbladder, and liver, which play essential roles in digestion.

Here's how these organs work together within your digestive system.

Mouth

The mouth is the beginning of the digestive tract. Digestion starts before you even take a bite-your salivary glands become active as soon as you see and smell a delicious dish, like pasta or warm bread. Once you start eating, you chew your food into smaller pieces for easier digestion. Your saliva mixes with the food, breaking it down into a form your body can absorb and use. When you swallow, your tongue pushes the food into your throat and esophagus.

Esophagus

The esophagus receives food from your mouth when you swallow. The epiglottis is a small flap that folds over your windpipe as you swallow to prevent you from choking (when food enters your windpipe). A series of muscular contractions within the esophagus, known as peristalsis, delivers food to your stomach.

But before reaching the stomach, the lower esophageal sphincter, a ring-like muscle at the bottom of your esophagus, relaxes to let the food in. It then contracts to prevent the stomach contents from flowing back into the esophagus. (When this muscle doesn't function properly and stomach contents flow back into the esophagus, you may experience acid reflux or heartburn.)

Stomach

The stomach is a hollow organ that holds food mixed with acid secreted by powerful enzyme-producing cells lining the stomach. The contents move through the digestive system with the help of hormones. Gastrin is a hormone produced in the stomach. It is produced by specialized cells called G-cells in the lining of the stomach and upper small intestine.

Gastrin:

1. **Stimulates Gastric Acid Release**: Gastrin signals your stomach to release **hydrochloric acid**, which aids in breaking down food during digestion.
2. **Promotes Muscle Contractions**: Gastrin stimulates muscle contractions in your stomach, contributing to gastric motility.
3. **Supports Stomach Lining Regeneration**: Gastrin helps your stomach lining (mucosa) replenish itself continuously.
4. **Coordinates Gallbladder and Pancreas**: Along with cholecystokinin, gastrin triggers the contraction of your gallbladder and pancreas, facilitating digestion.

Glucagon is a hormone produced in the alpha cells in the pancreas that helps regulate sugar levels. While insulin produced in the beta cells decreases elevated blood sugar levels, glucagon works in the opposite way, raising blood sugar when levels are too low (a condition known as hypoglycemia).

Small intestine

Made up of three segments — the duodenum, jejunum, and ileum — the small intestine is a 22-foot-long muscular tube that breaks down food using enzymes released by the pancreas and bile from the liver. Peristalsis also works in this organ, moving food through and mixing it with digestive juices from the pancreas and liver.

The duodenum, the first segment of the small intestine, is primarily responsible for the continuous breaking-down process of food. The jejunum and ileum, located lower in the intestine, are mainly responsible for the absorption of nutrients into the bloodstream.

The contents of the small intestine start as semi-solid and end in a liquid form after passing through the organ. The change in consistency is due to the action of water, bile, enzymes, and mucus. Once nutrients are absorbed, the remaining liquid food residue passes from the small intestine to the large intestine (colon).

Pancreas

The pancreas secretes digestive enzymes into the duodenum, breaking down protein, fats, and carbohydrates. The pancreas also produces insulin and glucagon, which are released directly into the bloodstream. Insulin is the chief hormone in your body that metabolizes sugar, while glucagon helps raise sugar levels when they are low.

Liver

The liver has many functions, but its primary role in the digestive system is to process the nutrients absorbed from the small intestine. Bile, a fluid released by the liver and secreted into the small intestine, also plays a vital role in digesting fat and certain vitamins.

The liver acts as your body's chemical "factory," transforming the raw materials absorbed from the intestine into chemicals your body needs to function.

The liver also detoxifies potentially harmful substances, breaking down and excreting various drugs and chemicals that could be toxic to your body.

Gallbladder

The gallbladder stores and concentrates bile produced by the liver. It then releases this bile into the duodenum of the small intestine to help in the absorption and digestion of fats.

Colon

The colon is responsible for processing waste, ensuring your bowel movements are easy and convenient. It's a 6-foot-long muscular tube that connects the small intestine to the rectum.

The colon includes the cecum, the ascending (right) colon, the transverse (across) colon, the descending (left) colon, and the sigmoid colon, which connects to the rectum.

Stool, or waste left over from digestion, is passed through the colon via peristalsis, beginning as a liquid and eventually becoming solid. As stool passes through the colon, water is absorbed. The stool accumulates in the sigmoid (S-shaped) colon until a "mass movement" empties it into the rectum once or twice daily.

It usually takes about 36 hours for stool to get through the colon. The stool mainly consists of food debris and beneficial bacteria known as probiotics. These "good" bacteria perform essential functions such as synthesizing vitamins, peptides, and chemicals for organs like the brain and establishing a gut-brain connection. When the descending colon fills with stool or feces, it empties its contents into the rectum, beginning the process of elimination (bowel movement).

Rectum

The rectum is an 8-inch, small chamber that connects the colon to the anus. Its function is to receive stool from the colon, signals you the need for evacuation (pooped out), and hold the stool until it is ready to be eliminated. When gas or stool enters the rectum, sensors send a message to the brain. The brain then decides the time to release the contents.

Once the brain gives the signals, the sphincters relax, and the rectum contracts disposing its contents. If the contents remain for any reason, the sphincter contracts and the rectum adjusts, causing the sensation to temporarily disappears until a convenient time for elimination.

Anus

The anus is the last part of the digestive tract. It is a 2-inch canal composed of the pelvic floor muscles and two anal sphincters (internal and external). The lining of the upper anus can detect rectal contents. It lets you know whether the contents are liquid, gas, or solid.

The pelvic floor muscles create an angle between the rectum and anus that prevents stool from coming out unintentionally. The internal sphincter is always tight, except when stool enters the rectum. This contracted internal sphincter keeps us continent (prevents us from pooping involuntarily) when we are asleep or unaware of the presence of stool.

When we feel the urge to go to the bathroom, we rely on our external sphincter to hold the stool until we reach the toilet. It then relaxes to release the contents.

What are some common conditions that affect the digestive system?

Both temporary conditions and long-term or chronic diseases and disorders affect the digestive system. It's common to experience issues such as constipation, diarrhea, or heartburn from time to time. However, if you frequently experience digestive issues like these, be sure to contact your healthcare professional. These symptoms could be a sign of a more severe disorder that requires medical attention and treatment.

Short-term or temporary conditions that affect the digestive system include:

- **Constipation:** Constipation generally happens when you go poop (have a bowel movement) less frequently than you usually do. When you're constipated, your poop is often dry, hard, and difficult or painful to pass.
- **Diarrhea**: Diarrhea happens when you have loose or watery poop. It can be caused by various factors, including bacterial infections, but sometimes the cause is unknown.

- **Heartburn**: Although it has "heart" in its name, heartburn is a digestive issue. Heartburn is an uncomfortable burning feeling in your chest that can move up your neck and throat. It occurs when acidic digestive juices from your stomach flow back into your esophagus.
- **Hemorrhoids**: Hemorrhoids are swollen veins located inside and outside of your anus and rectum. They can cause discomfort, pain, and rectal bleeding.
- **Stomach flu (gastroenteritis)**: Stomach flu is an infection of the stomach and upper part of the small intestine, often caused by a virus. It usually lasts less than a week, affecting millions of people every year.
- **Ulcers**: An ulcer is a sore that develops on the lining of the esophagus, stomach, or small intestine. The most common causes of ulcers are infection with a bacteria called Helicobacter pylori (H. pylori) and long-term use of anti-inflammatory drugs such as ibuprofen.
- **Gallstones:** Gallstones are small pieces of solid material formed from digestive fluid in your gallbladder, a small organ located beneath your liver.

Common digestive system diseases and disorders include:

- **GERD (Chronic Acid Reflux)**: Gastroesophageal reflux disease (GERD) is a condition that occurs when acid-containing contents in your stomach frequently leak back into your esophagus.
- **Peptic ulcers: Peptic ulcers develop** when areas of the stomach and the duodenum lose the protective mucous lining. The acid burns the tissues below, producing a chemical burn. If the area is not protected, the stomach or duodenum wall may perforate, causing a leak of food and acid into the abdominal cavity. This perforation is catastrophic and an emergency. Bacteria like Helicobacter Pylori may trigger an ulcer if left untreated.
- **Irritable bowel syndrome (IBS)**: IBS is a condition where the muscles of the colon contract irregularly. People with

IBS experiences excessive gas, abdominal pain, and cramps. Increased intestinal permeability secondary to dysbiosis usually occurs in chronic inflammatory conditions affecting the intestine.
- **Lactose intolerance**: People with lactose intolerance cannot digest lactose, a sugar primarily found in milk and dairy products.
- **Diverticulosis and diverticulitis**: Diverticulosis and diverticulitis are two conditions that occur in the large intestine (also called the colon). Both share the common feature of diverticula, which are pockets or bulges that form in the colon's wall.
- **Cancer**: Gastrointestinal (GI) cancers affect tissues and organs in the digestive system. There are multiple types of GI cancers. The most common include esophageal, gastric (stomach), colon and rectal (colorectal), pancreatic, and liver cancers.
- **Crohn's disease**: Crohn's disease is a lifelong form of inflammatory bowel disease (IBD) that causes irritation and inflammation throughout the digestive tract.
- **Celiac disease**: Celiac disease is an autoimmune disorder that can damage your small intestine. The damage happens when a person with celiac disease consumes gluten, wheat, barley, and rye protein. This condition is worsened when there is a "leaky gut," which allows harmful substances to pass through the intestinal lining.

What does the digestive system do?

Your digestive system transforms food into the nutrients and energy you need to survive. After processing, food is converted into solid waste, or stool, which is disposed of when you have a bowel movement. Eating right helps protect our gastrointestinal system and internal organs. Whereas eating the wrong foods is the cause of many degenerative diseases, cardiovascular problems, neurological disorders, anxiety, depression, cancer, premature aging, and reduced lifespan. We will explore these critical issues in the following sections.

Why is Digestion Important?

Digestion is important because your body needs nutrients from food and liquids to stay healthy and function properly. These nutrients include carbohydrates, proteins, fats, vitamins, minerals, and water. Your digestive system breaks down and absorbs the nutrients from the food and liquids you consume to provide energy, support growth, and repair cells.

As food moves through the digestive tract, it gradually changed its formuntil it is suitable for the circulatory system to absorb and deliver to its destination. This sensitive system may become upset if something irritates or triggers an inflammatory response. These common problems include heartburn, stomach ache, colic, bloating, chest pain, gas, diarrhea, constipation, vomiting, headaches, and brain fog.

Food is one of the greatest pleasures in life. Eating delicious food makes us feel energized, happy, and more vigorous. However, food can also make us sick and deplete our energyif the food we ingest doesn't agree with us for any reason. These reactions highlight how our gut is connected to our brain.

Our digestive system is also the host of trillions of guests—the microbiome—who, as dutiful servants, help us digest the food and produce chemicals necessary for vital functions. I will take you to the microbiome world to introduce you to the massive universe of living organisms working for us to help with our survival and health.

Is our gut connected to our brain?

Yes. There is a strong connection between our digestive system and our brain. The vagus nerve directly connects the brain to our digestive system, allowing signals to travel both ways

The gut-brain connection is complex and bidirectional. Signals pass both ways between your digestive system and central nervous system, meaning that one's health can affect the others. Key players in this connection include your enteric nervous system, the vagus nerve, and the gut microbiome.

Your brain communicates to your gut, and your gut communicates back. If you've ever had a "gut feeling," you've experienced this communication. It's how the thought of an exciting event can make you feel "butterflies in your stomach," while the idea of something dreadful might be "gut-wrenching." It is also how the feeling in your gut can influence your decision-making, as in "going with your gut." The cells lining the intestines have multiple connections to nerves in the intestinal wall, which carry information to the brain through the vagus nerve.

More information passes between your brain and your gut than any other body system. In fact, more nerve cells are in your gut than anywhere outside your brain.

What we eat is crucial to our overall health, and the types of food available have varied greatly throughout history, depending on what was available. Our brains and guts need to stay in close contact to ensure we receive the necessary nutrients. If we eat something harmful or are required to put the brakes on digestion, our body has developed a reliable alarm system.

This alarm system includes the emotional part of your brain. After a physical injury, your emotional brain kicks in to help you remember to avoid similar injuries in the future. Emotions can make physical sensations in your gut feel more intense. Intense physical sensations can increase your stress levels and your emotional response. This feedback loop between your brain and gut is powerful and constantly at work.

Studies suggest that the crosstalk between your gut and brain may influence:

- Hunger and satiety
- Food cravings
- Food sensitivities
- Gut motility (muscle movements)
- Digestion
- Metabolism

- Mood
- Behavior
- Stress levels
- Pain sensitivity
- Cognitive function
- Immunity

The gut-brain axis is the network of nerves that connect your brain and gut, allowing you to send signals back and forth. Additionally, your nervous system works closely with your endocrine system, producing hormones that regulate hunger, fullness, and stress. It works closely with your immune system to respond appropriately to injury or disease in your gut.

Within this network, some key players in the gut-brain connection include:

Enteric Nervous System

Your enteric nervous system is the neural network that operates within your gastrointestinal (GI) tract, controlling its digestive functions. With more than 500 million neurons, it's the most complex neural network outside your brain. It is unique because it can function independently from your brain and central nervous system, leading some scientists to refer to it as a "second brain."

I personally experienced the power of this system. In my early twenties, while a medical student and later as a resident, I developed a peptic ulcer in my duodenum, just outside of the stomach. At that time, there were no medicines available. The pain was excruciating and exacerbated by the anxiety of multiple tests, sleep deprivation, and coffee consumption. I adopted a diet free of citrus juices, spices, coffee, sodas, and alcoholic beverages. It worked. My brain guided me to eliminate many foods and chemicals affecting my intestine and overall health. Since then, I realized that my digestive system truly acts as my "second brain."

Your enteric nervous system is a special division of your autonomic nervous system that governs the automatic functions of your internal organs. While it operates as part of your overall autonomic nervous system, it can also act on its own. It can gather information about the conditions inside your GI tract, process it locally, and generate responses without sending it back to your brain.

Vagus Nerve

Your vagus nerve is the main link between your enteric nervous system and your brain. It is one of your 12 cranial nerves, which begin in your skull and travel down through your body, branching out along the way. Your vagus nerve conveys sensory information about the conditions inside your gut from your enteric nervous system to your brain. In response, it transmits motor signals from your brain to your gut.

The vagus nerve mediates various reflexes that operate within your gut in response to changing conditions, like chemical changes or the presence of food. These are called vagal reflexes. Intrinsic vagal reflexes operate within your enteric nervous system without involving your brain. On the other hand, extrinsic reflexes operate through communication between your enteric nervous system and central nervous system.

Gut Microbiome

Believe it or not, the bacteria in your gut also play a role in the gut-brain connection. Gut microbes produce or help in producing many chemical neurotransmitters, like dopamine and serotonin, which convey messages between your intestines and brain. They also make other chemicals that can affect your brain through your bloodstream. In turn, your brain and gut can affect your gut microbiome by altering its environment.

Recent studies have shown that the gut microbiome may be involved in neurological, mental health, and functional gastrointestinal disorders. Functional disorders cause persistent symptoms without any apparent physical cause. There is significant overlap among people with functional gastrointestinal disorders, such as IBS (Irritable Bowel Syndrome), and those with mental health disorders, like anxiety.

What Types of Medical Conditions or Symptoms Might Involve the Gut-Brain Axis?

Disorders related to the gut-brain axis may include:

- Irritable bowel syndrome
- Functional constipation or diarrhea
- Anxiety and depression
- Non-cardiac chest pain
- Infant colic
- Functional dyspepsia
- Functional dysphagia
- Gastroparesis
- Anismus
- Chronic stress
- Chronic fatigue
- Chronic pain
- Visceral hypersensitivity
- Obesity
- Autism
- Parkinson's Disease
- Multiple sclerosis

What Can I Do at Home to Nurture My Gut-Brain Axis?

The best way to take care of your gut health daily — and maybe improve your brain health— is by maintaining a healthy, balanced diet. Additionally, you can also care for your brain health — and maybe, through it, your gut health — by following my DRESS-SS prescription.

What type of diet is suitable for the gut-brain axis?

A good rule of thumb is to eat various whole foods, emphasizing plant-based foods. More diversity in your diet leads to a more diverse gut microbiome, which improves overall gut health. Whole foods and plants also provide more nutrition per calorie than processed foods, leaving less room for harmful additives, sweeteners, and saturated fats. Instead, they offer:

- Fiber. Most plants contain both types of fiber, which help regulate your bowel movements and feed the helpful microbiota inside. These microbes, in turn, nourish your gut lining.
- Prebiotics, Probiotics, and Postbiotics. Probiotics are the live bacteria in fermented foods, like yogurt and sauerkraut. Prebiotics are the fibers and complex starches that these bacteria feed on. Postbiotics are the metabolic by-products made by probiotics that have essential functions in the body and the health of the intestinal wall.
- Antioxidants. Antioxidants, which occur naturally in various fruits and vegetables, help fight free radicals in your body and prevent inflammation. Different foods contain different types of antioxidants.
- Anti-Inflammatory foods. A whole-food, plant-rich diet is naturally anti-inflammatory because it reduces the intake of sugar, additives, saturated fats, cholesterol, mycotoxins, and harmful chemicals added during the process. By eating right and adopting an anti-inflammatory diet, you will have a healthy microbiome, giving you better health and longevity.

In subsequent chapters, we will explore the importance of a plant-based diet and the microbiome.

CHAPTER 2

What is the microbiome?

The gut hosts trillions of residents with different DNA and structure. Billions of years ago, multicellular organisms lacked the means to process foods efficiently and produce enough energy for survival. Somehow, we made a trade and allowed different kinds of bacteria to become our guests if they could help us process our foods. Over time, this symbiotic relationship has allowed us to survive and thrive. This community of microorganisms is called the microbiome. The microbiota are the living members that form the microbiome. Some researchers consider the microbiome a newly discovered organ because of its profound impact on human health. The microbiome has a role in our health.

Different communities within the microbiome produce chemicals, or metabolites, that affect our health. Some of these chemicals are neurotransmitters that affect the function of our brains. Serotonin and dopamine are examples. The microbiome also plays a role in the development of autoimmune diseases. It forms a biofilm along the intestinal wall, protecting the intestinal lining. The gut bacteria promote homeostasis and decrease intestinal permeability; the biofilm collectively forms "ecological niches." However, inflammation decreases the thickness of the biofilm, increases intestinal permeability or leaky gut, and leads to autoimmune diseases. The gut lining produces more than 100 million neurotransmitters, similar to those in the central nervous system. This system is independent of the brain and can operate by its own; for this reason, it is also known as the "second brain". There is a close association between the gut and the brain through the vagus nerve, which his constitutes the gut-brain connection. The nerves along the intestine are known as the enteric nervous system (ENS).

Many brain diseases are linked to the enteric nervous system or the gut. Parkinson's is one of its examples. Deficiencies of dopamine in the brain can be associated with deficiencies in the gut. Lactobacillus Plantarum SP128 deficiency in the gut is associated with neurological degenerative disorders like Parkinson's. Destruction of this bacteria after administering antibiotics for an infection treated with oral antibiotics leads to many problems. The failure to restore this valuable probiotic leads to a decline in dopamine and serotonin. It is not unusual for people with a deficiency of this probiotic to begin to experience tremors, depression, and anxiety. Interestingly, brain lesions of Alzheimer's disease are also present in the enteric nervous system. (ENS)

Probiotics like Lactobacillus rhamnosus produce metabolites that affect the brain. A deficiency in this probiotic can lead to increased stress, anxiety, and depression. It is also present in the healthy female genito-urinary tract and is helpful in regaining control in cases of bacterial vaginosis and small intestinal bacterial overgrowth (SIBO).

What is a probiotic?

Probiotics (from the Latin word "probios,", meaning *for life*) are bacteria of human and nonhuman origin that improve health. Probiotics support life in the host as opposed to antibiotics that kill and destroy the microbiota. Many illnesses develop after treatments with antibiotics, which often destroy probiotics that promote health.

Fecal microbiota transplantation has proven more effective in treating infections caused by Clostridium difficile than the antibiotic vancomycin. Some probiotics from yeast are superior to those from bacterial origin. For example, Saccharomyces boulardii is a probiotic superior to Lactobacillus rhamnosus for treating persistent diarrhea in both children and adults.

Probiotics are our friends. A diet deficient in these microorganisms is not healthy. A good diet is not complete without a good balance of probiotics. Fermented foods are rich in healthy probiotics and should be part of our diet intake for a more balanced equilibrium.

What Drugs Affect the Balance of the Gut Microbiome?

Many drugs, mycotoxins, and certain foods can alter the balance of the microbiome populations.

The gut microbiome plays a crucial role in our overall health, including how our bodies respond to medications. Some drugs can destroy or interact with the gut microbiome:

1. Proton Pump Inhibitors (PPIs): These drugs treat dyspepsia (indigestion) and acid reflux. They affect and alter the microbiome population by increasing the abundance of bacteria.
2. Metformin: Metformin is a drug widely prescribed to manage Type 2 diabetes. It has been linked to higher levels of potentially harmful bacteria.
3. Antibiotics: Oral antibiotics for treating systemic bacterial infections cause extensive gut microbiome disruption, often leading to the loss of beneficial bacteria and the development of harmful bacteria.
4. Laxatives: Laxatives, used to treat and prevent constipation, it can remove trillions of bacteria causing loss of significant and helpful microbiome bacteria.

Remember, "maintaining a healthy gut microbiome is essential for overall well-being!"

The gut microbiota of PPI users showed an increased abundance of upper gastrointestinal tract bacteria and increased fatty acid production. In contrast, metformin users had higher levels of the potentially harmful bacteria Escherichia coli (E. coli).

Researchers have found that other drug categories were associated with significant changes in bacterial populations in the gut. The use of certain antidepressants (called SSRIs or Selective Serotonin Reuptake Inhibitors) by those with IBS was associated with an abundance of potentially harmful bacteria species like Eubacterium ramulus. The use of oral steroids was associated with high levels of methanogenic bacteria, which predispose individuals to obesity and an increase in body mass index (BMI). The extensive use of antibiotics promotes the development of harmful bacteria like Clostridium Difficilis. The loss of helpful bacteria leads to deficiencies of neurotransmitters, peptides, and many other chemicals necessary for optimal health. When there is a loss of valuable bacteria, it is essential to use probiotics to replace them as soon as possible. To find out about deficiencies of the valuable microbiome-bacteria, a stool analysis or GI mapping is necessary to correct such deficiencies. Refer to Appendix B for a list of laboratories that provide these services.

What is a Prebiotic?

Prebiotics are foods rich in fiber for the bacteria flora in our gut. Probiotics make their way to the colon, these bacteria; metabolize and ferment them, helping to create other compounds that improve our health. Short-chain fatty acids are one of the byproducts of intestinal organisms' transformation of prebiotics. These fatty acids help provide energy to colon cells, promote mucus production, prevent inflammation, and help protect the gut lining.

Prebiotics also:

- Help regulate bowel movements.
- Produce neurotransmitters that facilitate communication between your gut and brain to trigger mood changes and other processes.
- Stimulate your body to make hormones that aid in appetite, appetite suppression, and other functions.
- Help your bones mineralize and absorb calcium and phosphorus, improving bone density.

- Improve your immune system functions.
- Enhance your body's anti-inflammatory response.
- Increase the production of good bacteria and decrease harmful bacteria that cause disease.

Prebiotics boost the growth of pre-existing helpful bacteria aiding our intestinal flora in producing products or chemicals called postbiotics. Most of them are short-chain fatty acids (SCFA) These postbiotics are absorbed in the colon and circulate throughout our body, with some reaching our brain. Most postbiotics behave like hormones. Without fiber in the diet, our good bugs cannot make these beneficial chemicals or hormones. People who eat fiber live longer and healthier lives. Good health is another reason a fiber-rich diet is necessary for eating right. Fiber-rich intake leads to "successful aging," which is defined as the absence of disability, cognitive impairment, depression, respiratory symptoms, or chronic diseases. More than fifty randomized trials showed that prebiotics like fiber can significantly improve blood sugar, blood pressure, weight, and cholesterol levels.

People who consume plant-based foods rich in fiber tend to carry good bacteria, such as *Prevotella* species. In contrast, people who consume Westernized diets rich in animal foods are more likely to carry *Bacteroides* species.

Prevotella produces more short-chain fatty acids, which are anti-inflammatory and help prevent the development of colon cancer. People who consume animal diets have primarily Bacteroides and suffer more autoimmune disorders like Hashimoto Thyroiditis, multiple sclerosis, and type 1 diabetes.

In countries like rural sub-Saharan Africa, where plant-based diets are common, there is no incidence of these autoimmune diseases or colon cancer.

However, in the US, African Americans who primarily consume animal diets suffer a higher incidence of colon cancer. Switching from plant-based to animal-based diets can change the gut flora and vice versa within days.

Vegetarians have more good bacteria, like *Bifido* and *Lactobacillus*, and produce more butyrate, acetate, and short-chain fatty acids. This can result in less inflammation and an improved intestinal barrier.

Animal-based diets promote the growth of *Bilophila* bacteria, leading to a drop in short-chain fatty acids and a rise in toxic levels of dangerous metabolites like TMAO (triethylamine oxide). TMAO is responsible for plaque formation in mice and has been demonstrated in interventional trials in humans. It raises the odds of dying of a stroke by 67 percent and causes the platelets to become stickier, resulting in the formation of clots.

People who have high levels of this metabolite (TMAO) suffer more frequently from cardiovascular disease, high blood pressure, and high cholesterol and are at risk of heart attacks, strokes, and colon cancer. In a study of more than 30,000 people for five years, it was found out that high levels of TMAO were present in nearly 50 % of people with high mortality risks.

Where does this toxic TMAO come from?

TMAO is produced by harmful bacteria in the gut that consume choline (concentrated in eggs), lecithin (in supplements), or carnitine (abundant in meat and energy drinks). However, plant-based choline, like pistachios and Brussels sprouts, do not raise the levels of TMAO.

The best strategy is to prevent the growth of harmful bacteria that make TMAO. To memorize this toxic chemical, use the phrase "Time to Minimize Any Omnivorous."

Are Probiotics Present in Foods?

Yes, probiotics are present in many foods and are also available in dietary supplements.

Food. Many foods have good bacteria. However, these bacteria don't always survive strong stomach acids and may not be able to reach the gut to provide health. Other foods have probiotic strains that can survive digestion and reach the gut.

Whether a food truly has beneficial probiotics depends on the levels of good bacteria contained when eaten, whether the good bacteria can survive digestion, and whether those strains of bacteria can support your health.

These are a few foods that contain probiotics.

- dried beans and other legumes
- garlic
- asparagus
- onions
- leeks
- certain artichokes
- green bananas
- wheat

What Are the Most Common Probiotics used as Dietary Supplements?

Probiotics are available in various forms, as capsules, powders, liquids, and more. The wide variety of available products can make it challenging to determine which ones offer health benefits based on science.

Some of the best probiotic strains for health include:

Akkermansia Municiphila. Essential in many metabolic functions and immune responses in the intestinal wall. It protects against bacteria that damage the mucin layers in the intestinal wall and can cause people with type 2 diabetes, obesity, and premature aging.

Lactobacillus acidophilus. Balances potentially harmful bacteria that can otherwise grow in your gut due to illness or antibiotics. This probiotic has antioxidant properties, helps to prevent wrinkles, and has antimelanogenic effects.

Lactobacillus fermentum. This strain strengthens your immune system and prevents gastrointestinal and upper respiratory infections.

Lactobacillus casei/paracasei. Useful to ease inflammatory bowel disease, which causes cramping, abdominal pain, bloating, gas, diarrhea, or constipation). It also helps to protect the skin barrier, is antiallergic, anti-inflammatory in the airways, and is immunobiotic. It helps to prevent antibiotic-associated diarrhea (AAD) and *Clostridium difficile* infections. The best-documented strains include yogurts like Actimel or DanActive and Yakult of Japanese origin. The last one helps to improve bowel movements in those suffering from constipation and helps to support a healthy population flora.

Lactobacillus reuteri. Supports heart health by balancing cholesterol levels. It also reduces ulcer-causing bacteria and supports female urinary tract and vaginal health.

Lactobacillus Bulgaricus. Commonly found in yogurt, this strain supports good digestion, prevents diarrhea, and helps relieve symptoms of irritable bowel syndrome (IBS).

Lactobacillus rhamnosus (LR32). Found naturally in your gut, although you can eat foods or take supplements to increase its benefits. It helps relieve IBS symptoms, treat diarrhea, strengthen your gut health, and protect against cavities. It helps to digest sugars like lactose and increases the production of short-chain fatty acids (SCFA).

Lactobacillus plantarum. It stimulates your digestive system, fights off disease-causing bacteria, and helps your body produce vitamins. Lactobacillus plantarum 299v is very effective in improving the intestinal flora. Current knowledge about the role of L. plantarum 299v supports the treatment of selected diseases, such as cancer, irritable bowel syndrome (IBS), and Clostridium difficile infection. The immunomodulating properties of L. plantarum 299v include increased anti-inflammatory cytokines, which reduce the risk of cancer and improve the efficacy of regimens. The intake of L. plantarum 299v benefits IBS patients due to the normalization of stool and relief of abdominal pain, which significantly improves the quality of life of IBS patients. In addition, the intake of L. plantarum 299v prevents antibiotic-associated diarrhea from *Clostridium Difficile*.

Bifidobacterium longum ssp. Longum. It helps prevent inflammation and provides some protection from colon cancer, intestinal infections, inflammatory bowel diseases, and even depression.

Bifidobacterium longum ssp. Infantis. Helpful to treat bowel problems, eczema, vaginal yeast infections, lactose intolerance, and urinary tract infections.

Bifidobacterium breve (B632, BR03, Yakult). Beneficial to children and infants with colitis, diarrhea, celiac disease, and those undergoing chemotherapy. It also helps with constipation, and allergies.

Bifidobacterium bifidum. Helps manage your digestive system, improve IBS, and boost your immune system.

Bifidobacterium animalis ssp. Lactis. Helps prevent infection and produces vitamins and other essential chemicals in your body.

Saccharomyces boulardii. Removes toxin from bacteria, protects against intestinal infections, increases the production of short-chain fatty acids (SCFA), improves the secretion of IgA in the intestinal wall, and decreases the production of inflammatory cytokines.

A good probiotic must contain live and active bacterial culture, which should be indicated on the packaging. Pay close attention to colony-forming units (CFU), which tell you the number of bacterial cells you'll get in each dose.

A general recommendation is to choose probiotic products containing at least 1 billion colony-forming units containing the genus *Lactobacillus*, *Bifidobacterium*, *Bacillus*, or *Saccharomyces boulardii*, as these are some of the most researched probiotics. Even then, you may have to delve deeper, as each genus of bacteria encompasses numerous strains that produce different results.

To determine how many colony-forming units you need to help with a specific condition, you should speak to a doctor before starting probiotic supplements to ensure they're right for you.

Pay close attention to the label and be mindful of how to store your probiotics. Generally, you'd want to keep them refrigerated (and ensure the place you're buying them from does the same). Heat can kill off the microorganisms in your probiotics if they're not stored correctly.

You'll also have to pay close attention to the expiration date, as colony-forming units tend to decline over time, rendering them less helpful.

Also, look for encapsulated probiotics with a food source, such as inulin, so it has something to feed off of and remain viable while sitting on the shelf.

Some labeling can also be misleading. For example, yogurt contains two "starter" bacterial cultures — *Streptococcus thermophilus* and *Lactobacillus bulgaricus* — but these bacteria are often destroyed by your stomach acid and provide no beneficial probiotic effect.

While some people prefer probiotic supplements over foods; Dr. Cresci, an expert in probiotics and nutrition, suggests that probiotic-rich foods are a better option. In particular, fermented foods — Like kombucha (fermented black tea), sauerkraut (refrigerated, not shelf-stable), kimchi (made from fermented cabbage), tempeh, and miso (made from fermented soybeans) — provide a nourishing environment in which healthful bacteria thrive and release important byproducts such as short chain fatty acids and butyrate.

What is butyrate?

Butyrate is produced when good gut bacteria help break down the dietary fiber in your large intestine (colon). It's one of several short-chain fatty acids named for their chemical structure.

Dr. Cresci, who has studied butyrate for more than a decade, says "It's amazing how many beneficial things it does for the body.".

Butyrate is vital to digestive health as it provides the primary energy source for your colon cells; meeting about 70% of their energy needs. It may also offer other health benefits, including supporting your immune system, reducing inflammation, and preventing diseases like cancer.

You can promote butyrate production by consuming foods high in fermentable fiber. For excellent natural sources, eat a healthy diet rich in:

- Fruit.
- Legumes.
- Vegetables.
- Whole grains.
- Resistant starches (such as boiled potatoes and rice).

Research shows that butyrate can benefit gut health, but we need further investigation to fully understand how it works and whether it has other benefits. Butyrate could encourage weight loss, stabilize blood sugars, maintain or improve intestinal function, and protect against or help treat certain diseases.

Here are some benefits of butyrate for your body:

- Reduce inflammation

Studies have shown that butyrate supplements may decrease the severity of disease-causing (pathogenic) bacterial infection by reducing inflammation. Butyrate could help prevent potentially fatal conditions such as sepsis.

Researchers have also linked low levels of butyrate to an increased risk of inflammatory intestinal disease and colorectal cancer.

2. Relieve gastrointestinal conditions

Butyrate supports the gut barrier, preventing bacteria and other microbes from entering your bloodstream. A sodium butyrate supplement may help with irritable bowel syndrome (IBS), diverticulitis, and Crohn's disease.

One study found that 66 adults with irritable bowel syndrome (IBS) who took a daily dose of sodium butyrate reported less abdominal pain. In another study, 9 of 13 people with Crohn's disease experienced improved symptoms after taking butyric acid every day for eight weeks.

3. Reduce colon cancer risk

Other research shows that a diet high in dietary fiber encourages butyrate production and could help lower your risk of colon cancer.

A laboratory study in human cancer cell lines found that sodium butyrate stopped the growth of colorectal cancer cells and caused cancer cell death (known as apoptosis). It also helps reduce damage caused by cancer or chemotherapy.

4. Increase insulin sensitivity

People with Type 2 diabetes often experience insulin resistance and obesity. Butyrate helps produce gut hormones that regulate blood sugar levels, potentially improving these symptoms. One study showed a potential link between butyrate production and lower insulin resistance.

5. Protect your brain

Butyrate-friendly foods and supplements may improve brain health. Research has shown that butyrate can protect your brain and improve its ability to adapt (plasticity).

Early studies suggest it may help prevent or treat conditions like stroke, depression, Parkinson's disease, and Alzheimer's disease.

6. Treat cardiovascular disease

Some studies suggest that butyrate may help protect your body against widespread cardiovascular diseases. Heart and blood vessel problems can increase your risk of:

- Atherosclerosis
- Heart failure
- High blood pressure
- Stroke

Enhance sleep. Butyrate's promise is to extend to your bedroom. Emerging evidence suggests that gut bacteria are a source of signals that promote sleep.

A 2019 study showed that mice and rats receiving butyrate increased non-rapid-eye movement (NREM) sleep for four hours after treatment. NREM includes essential stages of sleep that contribute to both physical and mental health.

Prebiotic foods

Prebiotic foods are typically high in certain types of fermentable soluble fiber. How you cook your food determines how many Prebiotics are available because your food changes composition based on how you cook it (or not cook it). Although there are many Prebiotics, three of the most common are resistant starches, inulin, and pectin.

Like fiber, resistant starches resist digestion and become a primary food source for microorganisms in your colon. When resistant starches break down, they often produce butyrate, which helps with water and electrolyte absorption, immune system functionality, and anti-inflammation.

Take potatoes, for example. Baking potatoes produce less resistant starch, but if you boil them and let them chill, the white, starchy film that forms is the resistant starch you want. When cooked food is rapidly cooled, its starches reorganize in a chemical process called retrogradation. The starches in this fiber resist digestion, and about 30 to 50 percent are not absorbed. Freezing bread before eating decreases the glycemic index, helping reduce blood sugar and insulin levels. Studies suggest that resistant starch also helps your microbiome to thrive. When carbohydrates break down and ferment to create resistant starch, they produce short-chain fatty acids like butyrate. This fatty acid is a great way to nourish your microbiome.

Resistant starches are present in the foods listed below; chill them after cooking or keep them in the refrigerator as leftovers for the following day.

- Boiled and chilled potatoes.
- Green bananas.
- Barley.
- Oats.
- Rice.
- Beans.
- Legumes.

Inulin is a prebiotic fiber found in many plants. This prebiotic can give you a feeling of fullness for extended periods, helping prevent overeating and promoting regular bowel movements. It can also help lower LDL (bad cholesterol), stabilize blood sugar levels, and increase the good bacteria in your gut. It may also help reduce the risk of colon cancer. While you can take inulin as a supplement in gummies, tablets, capsules, and powder form, foods high in inulin also tend to have additional benefits by providing antioxidants and other vitamins. Some of those foods high in inulin include:

- Asparagus.
- Burdock root.
- Chicory root.
- Dandelion greens.
- Garlic.
- Jerusalem artichokes.
- Leeks.
- Onions.
- Soybeans.
- Wild yams.

Pectin

Pectin is found in many fruits, especially in the pulp of raw apples. It is a gel-like starch often used to make jams and jelly. This starch has antioxidant and anti-tumor properties. It may also enhance the cells of your intestinal lining, decrease the ability for bacterial diseases to take hold, and improve the diversity of microorganisms in your gut. More human studies are needed to determine other beneficial results.

Foods high in pectin include:

- Apples.
- Apricots.
- Carrots.
- Green beans.
- Peaches.
- Raspberries.
- Tomatoes.
- Potatoes.

It's best if you introduce prebiotics into your diet gradually. Taking too much can cause too much gas and make you feel so bloated.

Prebiotics work best when taken during the day and not at night or late in the evening. Remember that fiber is good for you, and when you eat fiber, you get Prebiotics.

Is a Good Diet Alone the Final Answer for Good Health?

A good diet includes essential nutrients, prebiotics, probiotics, vitamins, minerals, and supplements. Most people never think about the microbiome, probiotics, or healthy bacteria as part of their diets for better nutrition, health, and longevity. However, someone has to help process these nutrients, and probiotics serve as our dutiful agents. You must take care of them and prevent their destruction with antibiotics or harmful bacteria.

Our digestive system is like a master chemistry engineer and guardian. Bacteria are the dutiful assistants and helpers. But this master guardian is under our control. This friendly guardian must process everything that enters our mouths, whether it is beneficial or harmful to our well-being and survival. Sometimes, when the guardian is furious and detects harmful bacteria coming in, it reacts with toxic substances that make us sick. We may experience heartburn, stomach aches, nausea, vomiting, or diarrhea shortly after consuming something. In these moments, we realize that we've eaten something wrong and need to take action to relieve symptoms and prevent dehydration or death.

Unfortunately, many people do not understand the importance of consuming healthy foods and nutrients to improve health and longevity.

Many eat almost anything without considering whether the food is nutritional or appropriate for our well-being and the processing by the healthy bacteria in our gut.

Many eat unhealthy foods, which in the common language is called "junk food." Junk food is not different than garbage food. Many turn their digestive system into trash disposals by consuming anything regardless of the quality of the food and the damage it may cause. It is difficult to separate the garbage when our food industry constantly adds additives and harmful chemicals to our food. The majority of processed foods fit this category. Many foods often contain insecticides, hormones, antibiotics, dangerous chemicals, toxic substances, and molds. They are also rich in harmful animal fats, sugars, and carbohydrates.

Many of these foods contain antibiotics that kill the good bacteria that help process the food and create vitamins and peptides to support all the cells in our bodies. The same goes with hormones: many industries give animals hormones to increase their size, and these hormones are passed to humans, causing imbalances in our endocrine system. Fish may be contaminated with mercury or heavy metals, which can harm pregnant women and their babies. Fish farms let the water where they raise fish have high levels of bacteria. Farmed fish eat grains, soy, and other harmful nutrients they can't process. To survive, they develop mechanisms to digest this unhealthy food. Farm fish contains high levels of harmful saturated fats derived from ARA, arachidonic acid, and bacteria. Getting oysters obtained from polluted waters can carry dangerous bacteria. The use of insecticides and weed killers is constant. Food like fruits and vegetables sometimes contain these chemicals in the skin or surface. Many food-processing plants don't care about our well-being as long as they can profit.

To stay healthy and protect our families, we must be aware of these practices to stay healthy and protect our families. Fresh, organic foods are a better choice and processed foods should be avoided as much as possible.

Why do we eat junk food when we know it is harmful?

People are often brainwashed since to believe that junk food is acceptable. The delusional thinking promoted by the food industry that junk food is good is despicable, all in pursuit of profits. Unfortunately, our governments and politicians accept campaign money from these companies and, in turn, allowing food processors and manufacturers to add harmful chemicals to our foods.

Parents also don't realize the damage they are doing to their children. Frequently, they feed their children too many carbs and sugars when they give sugary juices to infants and young children. They also reward children with ice cream, pizza, and sodas containing hundreds of grams of sugars, including harmful types like fructose found in syrups. No wonder why we see so many children becoming obese at an early age.

The same happens to many adults. They gain weight and are always looking for diets to lose weight. The advertisement for diets to lose weight and unregulated supplements is constant and deceptive. Ozempic is a popular drug that brings billions to the manufacturer to help control appetite. But what happens if people stop using this drug? The reality is weight loss and increased appetite returns. Why not start eating the right foods and avoid becoming dependent on an expensive drug? What is happening is that people are becoming addicted to a drug with no end in sight. You now understand why I am so critical of what medical education is doing to our doctors. The profession has become more of a form of drug pushers rather than honest doctors using good nutrients to prevent obesity and other harmful diseases. It is apparent people are concerned about their weight and health. Despite so many commercials, they may lose some pounds initially to regain the weight again when they stop their diets or drugs like Ozempic.

This book is our effort to contribute and help remove the clutter that causes confusion and discourages anyone with conflicting information. As a doctor with more than fifty years of experience, I encourage you to reflect on my wife and me as examples. In our first book, *Living Longer and Reversing Aging*, we explain why we look healthier and younger. This book is an expansion of what we already explained before. We are bringing updated information from renowned scientists and analyzing what is best and practical. Eating healthy foods prevents many of the degenerative diseases and premature deaths. We must learn to eat the right foods and educate ourselves and our children to ensure a longer, healthier life.

What Is a LeakyGut?

To add insult to injury, the delicate lining in our intestine may become more permeable, allowing harmful foods or undigested particles and bacteria to pass to our circulatory system, reaching our bloodstream where they don't belong. This condition is known as leaky gut syndrome.

Many of the symptoms we described before are present when the lining of the intestine is damaged, allowing more permeability along the intestine. The cells forming the intestinal lining are packed closely together and don't allow large particles to enter the bloodstream. Sometimes, they separate, creating a tiny hole that allows harmful particles or bacteria to enter the bloodstream. You can imagine the immediate reaction by our immune system. The white cells, acting as the border patrol, begin attacking by swallowing these particles or bacteria to destroy the enemy. If particles or bacteria are too large, they call for reinforcements. T cells and natural killer cells may come into action. The result is an inflammatory response characterized by the production of cytokines. Allergenic foods, like gluten, can trigger a similar reaction, such as an inflammatory response, when someone is sensitive to certain foods. Gluten causes Celiac disease. Removing gluten improves this condition. When a person has food sensitivities, the cells lining the intestinal wall release a protein named zonulin. The presence of this protein is a marker of inflammation at the intestinal wall level and is known as a "leaky gut."

High zonulin levels are present in many inflammatory conditions like Inflammatory Bowel Syndrome (IBS), Hashimoto's thyroiditis, type 1 diabetes, pancreatic cancer, ovarian cancer, glioma, multiple sclerosis, and many forms of mental illness, like schizophrenia and autism.

The same happens for autoimmune diseases. Most people with some degree of leaky gut suffer from chronic inflammation. People may be unaware of this syndrome, but it is a silent and destructive killer responsible for many illnesses and most degenerative diseases common as we age. There is currently intensive interest and research in understanding how this increased permeability leads to many diseases affecting humanity. Breaching the security of this border by undesirable bacteria or toxic substances puts our health, life, and happiness in danger. Securing and protecting this boundary should be the best approach to treating many illnesses. Unfortunately, most doctors are not interested or lack the knowledge to address the source of the problem and prefer to treat or manage a problem after a crash or illness develops. This sickness approach is one of the greatest mistakes of current medical education. Identifying the source prevents morbidity and the need for medications.

Fortunately, some doctors understand these issues and address the source. Some laboratories today offer specialized tests to determine if you have a leaky gut, food sensitivities, or an imbalanced microbiome.

The particles and bacteria that enter the bloodstream act as antigens, activating the T cells' production of antibodies. Zonulin and Occludin are proteins released by the cells lining the gut that open the gates and allow fluids to move back and forth along the intestinal membrane. These two proteins control the permeability of our gut. When elevated, these two proteins indicate damage to the tiny junctions between the cells in the intestine's lining. Also, lipopolysaccharides (LPS) antibodies outside the digestive system and detected in blood samples indicate a leaky gut. LPS are materials or remnants from the wall of bacteria in the blood after the white cells destroy them.

Larazotide is a pharmacological agent developed to inhibit zonulin production and tighten the junctions that allow increased intestinal permeability. These pharmaceuticals are helpful in cases of severe inflammatory response. Ideally, by eliminating the offending agent, the inflammatory response stops. Gluten is an example. The challenge is to find out all the foods that cause sensitivity and promote a leaky gut. We will discuss some of this testing ahead

Which Foods Cause a Leaky Gut?

If you have a food sensitivity, you likely have a leaky gut. There is always a silent inflammatory response, or "fire in your belly," anytime cytokines are produced in response to such sensitivities. This "fire" may become serious if you are highly sensitive to the food. Sensitivity to certain foods triggers the production of AG antibodies. Special blood tests to detect AG antibodies specific to foods are available through specialized laboratories. In our Appendix, I provide information on laboratories performing these tests. Eliminating the food responsible for the sensitivity eliminates the inflammatory response. Millions of people have food sensitivities and leaky gut, contributing to a chronic inflammatory syndrome. When too many cytokines are circulating, an individual who develops an infection like COVID-19 or receives a vaccine may experience a cytokine storm and become very sick. Many people who became seriously ill with COVID-19 or had a severe reaction to the vaccine likely had elevated cytokine levels from an autoimmune disease or a chronic inflammatory response in the gut.

The Most Common Foods Responsible for a Leaky Gut Are:

1) Sugar and Carbohydrates. Fructose is a sugar that the liver cannot fully digest and metabolize. It is the main ingredient of many syrups and it turns into fat in the liver and abdomen. Excess fat deposits in the liver lead to non-alcoholic fatty liver disease. People who consume too much sugar often develop insulin resistance and metabolic syndrome, and they are likely to become obese. The damage to the liver is similar to the damage done by consuming too much alcohol. Cirrhosis of the liver is a fatal disease that could be associated with liver cancer and premature death due to liver failure. Sugar is the preferred food of harmful bacteria, and their growth increases gut permeability, aggravating a leaky gut. Sugar also raises the production of AGEs (Advanced Glycation End products), which cause inflammation of arterial vessels, leading to atherosclerosis, Alzheimer's, and many chronic degenerative diseases. Artificial sweeteners also contribute to a leaky gut, and some can be very toxic. Aspartame has been linked to multiple myeloma despite denials from the manufacturer. Sucralose and other alternatives damage the lining of the intestine and harm healthy bacteria. White bread contains gluten and is rich in carbohydrates. No wonder people gain weight when eating bread or starchy foods every day. They also contribute to the elevation of blood sugar and the development of diabetes.
2) Alcohol. We have already discussed the effects on the liver and the development of cirrhosis. A glass of wine or a single beer won't damage your liver in one day, but significant consumption day after day can damage the liver and increase gut permeability.
3) Diary. Many people have been sensitive to dairy products since childhood. Some suffer from lactase deficiency, which causes the sugar lactose in milk to lead to diarrhea and

cramps. The symptoms are the result of an inflammatory response in the intestinal wall. Most cheeses, especially processed cheeses, contain added flavors. Milk from grass-fed animals is best. 2% milk or skim milk is better than whole milk if you already have elevated cholesterol and coronary heart disease. Milk is rich in sugars that contribute to inflammation and weight gain.

4) Animal Fats and Vegetable Oils are Rich in Saturated fats. Many vegetable oils contain omega-6, which is inflammatory. Anyone with chronic inflammation, coronary heart disease, or obesity should avoid vegetable oils from corn, sunflower, cottonseed, safflower, canola, and soy. Margarine and spreads with hydrogenated oils are rich in trans fats, which damage the arteries and promote plaque formation. Clarified ghee may be an alternative when combined with olive oil.

5) Fatty meats. Most meats are rich in inflammatory animal fats, leading to elevated cholesterol and VLDL. Overcooked meat is toxic to the lining of the colon. Most world health and professional organizations advise against eating overcooked meat as it can lead to the development of colon cancer. Burgers, hot dogs, bacon, and bologna are highly inflammatory and rich in animal fats, which are responsible for the obstruction of coronary arteries and lead to strokes. Avoid these foods all the time, as they are very toxic and shorten your healthspan and lifespan.

6) Processed Foods. They are rich in omega-6 and fats from hydrogenated plant oils, which may contribute to chronic kidney disease. They are present in many snacks, cereals, breads, and junk foods. French fries are one of the most toxic foods available. Fried in reheated oils rich in trans and kept at high temperatures for long periods, they are deadly. Fries have lots of harmful oils, AGEs, and carbohydrates. Cereals often contain added sugars, making them highly inflammatory and destructive to the microbiome.

7) Soy. This food is a plant phytoestrogen that affects the endocrine system, disrupting the hormone balance necessary for optimal health. Soy often contains pesticides that lead to toxicity, leaky gut, and chronic inflammation.
8) Legumes (Beans, Lentils, and Peanuts. These foods contain lectins and can be allergenic. Peanuts, in particular, can cause anaphylactic shock and death. A blood test to check for AG antibodies to peanuts is essential to prevent catastrophic events.

How Does Diet Play a Role in Chronic Inflammation?

Diet plays a crucial role in the development of chronic inflammation. Consuming saturated fat increases pro-inflammatory markers, particularly in diabetics and overweight individuals. However, this can affect anyone, regardless of genetic predisposition. Synthetic trans fats in hydrogenated oils increase inflammatory markers, specifically IL-6 and TNF-alpha, in overweight individuals. Overheated oils, commonly used every day in fast food chains and restaurants, can damage your body, increase the risk of obesity, and harm your arteries. Unfortunately, many people are unaware of this fact, contributing to millions of cases of cardiovascular disease, obesity, and cancer.

Consequently, we see an increase in inflammation-related diseases such as heart disease, atherosclerosis, heart attacks, obesity, diabetes, and cancer. To protect your health, it is essential to take steps to prevent chronic inflammation and the damage it causes to your arteries and organs by limiting the consumption of saturated fats as much as possible. An anti-inflammatory and calorie-restricted diet can significantly reduce the risk of developing chronic inflammation, which often begins with a leaky gut. Inflammation is the common factor behind the development of many chronic diseases as we age. Preventing chronic inflammation can reduce the onset of these illnesses and improve overall health and longevity.

What Are the Best Foods for a Healthy Gut and Microbiome?

Select anti-inflammatory foods. In general, an anti-inflammatory diet is beneficial in preventing chronic inflammation. Millions of people are unaware of food sensitivities that make them sick and contribute to obesity. Many diets involving foods rich in carbohydrates don't work. While people may lose weight initially, they often regain it after discontinuing the diet. These diets don't help because they ignore what happens to the microbiome.

1) Fruits with Low Glycemic Index. Many fruits contain complex sugars, including fructose. It's best to avoid fruits high in fructose as much as possible. Instead, opt for fruits rich in antioxidants and polyphenols as they are healthier and better—like most berries, including blueberries, raspberries, blackberries, and strawberries. The darker the color, the better. These fruits help fight cancer, slow cognitive decline, and reduce the risk of cardiovascular disease. One cup of berries daily protects against free radicals that damage your DNA.
2) Good Vegetable Oils. Avocado oil and olive oil are safe and protective, and excellent for cooking. Foods rich in omega-3 are excellent for nourishing the microbiome. Good bacteria thrive with omega-3. Fish is rich in omega 3, making fish, particularly wild salmon, a good source of protein and healthy fats. Nuts like almonds and walnuts are also high in omega-3 fatty acids, fiber, and proteins Avoid farmed fish, which tends to be rich in saturated fats. This recommendation also applies to farmed salmon.
3) Leafy Greens. Most green vegetables are rich in polyphenols and antioxidants, which are anti-inflammatory flavonoids that help to restore cellular health. As a rule, the darker the color, the more nutritious the greens. They are also rich in vitamins A, C, and K. Broccoli is particularly rich in potassium and magnesium, making it one of the best anti-inflammatory foods. Other similar greens include cabbage,

cauliflower, and Brussels sprouts, all of which help reduce oxidative stress.
5) Fish, Salmon, and Hormone-Free Poultry. Wild salmon is better than farm-raised or Atlantic salmon. Wild salmon is rich in omega-3 fatty acids, which protect and help the microbiome produce vitamins and peptides. It is also a good source of proteins and contains all essential amino acids for cellular growth.
6) Probiotics. Bacteria and some yeasts have been residents of our digestive system for millions of years. These microorganisms help to digest and metabolize foods by fermentation. Most of them belong to the Lactobacillus and Bifidobacterium families. Saccharomyces boulardii is a fungus well known for its positive results in patients with inflammation. These probiotics help to produce beneficial metabolites, peptides, ácido linoleic, secondary biliary acids, vitamin K, and B vitamins such as thiamine, riboflavin, pantothenic acid, pyridoxine, biotin, folic acid, cobalamin (B12). They also help the production of IgA antibodies and antimicrobial peptides, reduce toxins, and help maintain the integrity of the intestinal lining. Probiotics help regulate the immune system and antioxidant systems. A list of valuable probiotic strains is provided ahead.
7) Prebiotics. Prebiotics include fiber and non-digestible foods that help the microbiome grow and perform positive functions to allow the body to metabolize and produce chemicals unavailable in our diets. Fermented foods like sauerkraut, kimchi, coconut kefir, kombucha, pickled vegetables, pickled beets, and olives enhance the microbiome's work.

Can Probiotics Replace Many Synthetic Drugs?

Yes. Many companies are developing probiotic strains capable of producing hormones, neurotransmitters, peptides, and anticancer chemicals. Psychobiotics, immunobiotics, and oncobiotics are advancing to a point where probiotics can make these chemicals without the need for regular prescription medications.

Currently, some labs are producing modified probiotics using splicing techniques like CRISPR to make them more specific in treating certain conditions or illnesses. Some new probiotics help prevent gestational diabetes or eczemas and may have other therapeutic uses. They are known as "live biotherapeutic products" (LBPs) in the US. These advances are not new, but they attempt to replace harmful microbes with beneficial microbes. Used as a drug, LBPs require medical supervision since they treat specific conditions.

Psychobiotics modulate the gut-brain connection to improve mental health and neurodegenerative diseases. Immunobiotics affect T cells to improve autoimmune diseases. Oncobiotics are probiotics that help in the prevention and treatment of cancers. The field of pharmabiotics is growing, offering precision medicine to treat various illnesses.

What Are Synbiotics?

Synbiotics are mixtures of probiotics (helpful gut bacteria) and prebiotics (non-digestible fibers that help these bacteria grow). Specifically, they are combinations of these two components that work together (synergistically) in your digestive tract.

The idea behind synbiotics is that the prebiotics help the probiotics survive in your intestines. Synbiotics can help balance your gut bacteria and benefit your health, metabolism, and immune system.

You can get synbiotics as supplements or in foods. Researchers have added them to pasta, beverages, candy, and yogurt

How Do You Test for Leaky Gut and Food Sensitivity?

Your doctor should be familiar with these critical tests and their interpretation. However, many doctors are unfamiliar with these tests and lack experience in diagnosing and treating leaky gut and its consequences. Gastroenterologists and Functional Medicine doctors understand how a leaky gut could be the source of many of your symptoms.

As a general guideline, keep a diary of what you eat, noting what happens when you wake up and before you go to bed. Highlight foods that don't agree with you. Make notes of symptoms like heartburn, stomach ache, flatulence, diarrhea, headaches, brain fog, joint or muscle pains, etc. By doing this, you become a detective helping your doctor to find the cause.

Your doctor may request some basic test to start:

1. Complete Blood Count (CBC).
2. Comprehensive Metabolic Panel (CMP).
3. Lipid panel, including HDL, LDL (A and B form), triglycerides, lipoprotein A and B, or Apo A and Apo B.
4. Homocysteine levels.
5. Vitamin D3 levels.
6. Magnesium levels.
7. Thyroid panel (Free T3, T4).
8. Zonulin, Occludin, and LPS levels.
9. GI map. This stool sample test helps identify pathological and good bacteria, fungi, and parasites in your microbiome.
10. Food Sensitivity Test. Some labs identify over 250 food sensitivities with a small blood sample using a simple at-home collection kit provided by the lab. Evaluation for IgG and IgE antibodies is best. They measure IgG1-4 with complement activation via marker C3d as a marker of inflammation.
11. Mycotoxin test to assess for toxins and molds. Most labs provide kits to collect samples.
12. Additional inflammation markers: Hs CRP, Sed Rate, IL-6, and TNF-alpha.

Once the results are available, your doctor will explain what is wrong with your microbiome. With the help of an experienced nutritionist familiar with food sensitivities and leaky gut, they should provide a plan of action. Removing the antigenic foods responsible for the highest levels of inflammation is the first step. It would help to remember that the immune system doesn't forget its "enemies" T and B cells have mechanisms to recall antigens in the food that trigger an inflammatory response. Your doctor may recommend probiotics necessary to improve the intestinal flora for better protection of the intestinal wall and digestion of foods. He may start antibiotic treatment to eliminate dangerous bacteria if pathogenic bacteria are present. Treatment with antibiotics is generally short, except in cases of infections by Helicobacter Pylori. You may need to adopt dietary changes for the rest of your life. Follow-up testing may be necessary in six months to assess progress.

What Is the Best Diet to Follow?

Intermittent fasting combined with a plant-based diet is the best to stay healthy and reduce biological age. If you have food sensitivities, you should follow an anti-inflammatory diet based on sensitivity testing, as some plant foods may cause sensitivities and contribute to a leaky gut. A food sensitivity test can help identify these problematic foods.

In my opinion, as I've recommended before, an anti-inflammatory diet- which is essentially a vegan diet- is best for someone with chronic inflammatory problems and autoimmune diseases, provided they have no food sensitivities or elevated markers of inflammation. Zonulin is an essential marker of intestinal permeability. If this marker is elevated, you should undergo food sensitivity testing. This diet is also suitable for anyone who doesn't have any inflammatory issues.

Intermittent fasting is essential if you want to lose or maintain your weight. Recent studies in mice have shown additional benefits of the FMD (Fasting Mimicking Diets), reducing the risk of age-related diseases like cancer, heart disease, and diabetes, according to Dr. Longo, a nutrition expert.

The anti-inflammatory diet is also ideal for people with fibromyalgia and chronic inflammatory syndrome.

Symptoms of fibromyalgia are usually related to food sensitivities and chronic gut inflammation.

With proper microbiome mapping and food sensitivity testing, you should, with the help of a doctor or a nutritionist, develop a new microbiome to eliminate your symptoms.

You can eliminate most food sensitivities by identifying specific IgG antibodies. Any testing should include screening for mycotoxins, which are prevalent in many foods. Frequently, toxins from molds can grow in grains, coffee beans, and corn before processing and are present in bread, flour, and many food products. The mold's toxins stay throughout the entire process until consumed, triggering an inflammatory response in your microbiome or intestinal cells.

Akkermansia Municiphila is an excellent probiotic to add to your new microbiome. It helps protect the intestinal wall by increasing the mucin levels.

I recommend seeking professional help from a gastroenterologist or a doctor who specializes in functional medicine to guide you in developing a new intestinal flora. An anti-inflammatory diet serves as a good foundation for an everyday diet because it prevents chronic inflammation, which is the common denominator of many cardiovascular diseases, autoimmune disorders, Alzheimer's, and cancer.

Vegan diets are also an excellent baseline to prevent the development of many inflammatory conditions, obesity, and cardiovascular disease. I prefer a modified vegan diet for everyday meals.

A good diet should include proteins, healthy fats like polyunsaturated fats from extra virgin olive oil and avocado oil, omega-3 in wild salmon, and foods containing vitamin B complex, such as B12, folic acid, along with low carbs and resistant starches. Sugars and carbs should be limited to no more than 30 gm a day, unless you are a growing child or who requires more carbohydrates due to the higher level of activities and exercise. Avoid sodas and fruit juices, as they contain high sugar levels. I don't recommend meats of any kind, dairy, or eggs, as these foods promote cardiovascular disease.

Dr. Esselstyn reversed plaque formation in patients with severe coronary disease by eliminating these foods from their diets (see the section "Diets to End Coronary Artery Disease and Atherosclerosis" in Chapter 3.

To keep your weight down, you should practice intermittent fasting. Sixteen hours of fasting and only eight hours of eating a balanced diet will help you to increase your AMPK levels. As we have emphasized, low-calorie intake promotes health and longevity.

Any diet should include a healthy amount of antioxidants. My favorites are blue fruits, such as blueberries, blackberries, cranberries, raspberries, strawberries, cherries, plums, and apples.

When choosing fruit, look for those with a low glycemic index, since they don't raise your blood sugar levels too quickly. A good diet should contain enough fiber and resistant starches to counter the effects of elevated blood sugar spikes. Fiber slows down the absorption of carbs, and a plant-based diet is rich in fiber. Remember to eat right every day.. A healthy diet is the foundation for living healthier and achieving old age with energy, vitality, and excellent cognition. Many diseases seen in aging populations are preventable. If you want to stay in great shape as you age, looking young and healthy, you should start early and not wait until you've experienced significant health decline.

Table 1 lists foods rich in antioxidants. For low-carb foods, please check Table 2.

For B complex vitamins, check Table 3.

CHAPTER 3

How Can a Balanced Diet Improve Your Health and Quality of Life?

"Don't sacrifice greater happiness for minor happiness."

The words of wisdom by the Ancient Greek philosopher Epicurus of Samos, whichopened this chapter, have guided me throughout my life, helping me achieve success and greater happiness. Eating is one of the greatest pleasures in life, but eating the wrong food or eating in excess can cause harm.

Junk foods and sugary drinks may provide immediate gratification, but over time, they will cause harm. Children raised on harmful diets that include these dangerous foods will eventually develop diabetes or heart disease, or die prematurely as adults. Eating the right food as we grow up is better than suffering illness or premature death later in life. Chronic inflammation is the common thread responsible for many diseases, short lifespans, and premature deaths. I emphasize anti-inflammatory diets as the best way to live free of pain, illness, and disability.

This chapter will cover diets, including the diets we follow, reasons why many diets fail, inflammatory diets, DNA methylation, sugar addiction, obesity, and free radicals as a cause of cancer. We will continue with vitamins, minerals, and supplements in another chapter for more detail. Since personal health plays a crucial role in these pursuits, we must first address diet and nutrients essential for a healthy lifestyle, and examine how nutrients and free radicals may affect our chromosomes and mitochondria at the cellular level.

Most people understand that food is one of the essential elements necessary to stay alive. Poor nutrition is detrimental to our health and leads to nutritional deficiencies at the cellular level and in supportive tissues, which can cause serious health consequences.

We have evolved over millions of years, and our humanoid ancestors mainly ate plant-based foods. With civilization, we have modified our diets and created thousands of processed foods containing many ingredients harmful to our cells and organs. The introduction of refined sugar into our diets has been a curse rather than a blessing. Most cases of diabetes, chronic inflammatory diseases, and cancers have developed or become more apparent with a diet rich in sugars. Sugar is addictive, has shortened our lifespan, and has caused numerous health problems. Animals don't depend on sugars for their survival. They can't refine sugars, which are detrimental to both animals and humans. The fact that many animals are herbivores and never consume sugars or saturated animal fats proves that these foods are unnecessary for survival. We don't need extensive studies to verify these facts; we can observe nature and realize that a plant-based diet is key to survival and good health. Another nutrient not present in our ancestors' diets is animal saturated fats. The consumption and preparation of meat, poultry, and processed foods containing saturated fats are responsible for the extensive formation of plaques in our arteries, which lead to heart attacks and strokes, decimating millions of people for centuries.

In his book "How Not to Age," Dr. Michael Greger proposes returning to nature. "Given that the healthiest foods tend to come from plants, it should be no surprise that healthy plant-based diets are associated with a lower risk of premature death in the general population and, specifically, among older adults," he says.

Dan Buettner, the founder of the Blue Zones organization and author of many books researching areas where people enjoy long and healthy lives, found several common characteristics among these populations. After several dietary surveys, his group discovered that plant-based foods are their primary nutrition source. His organization created food guidelines to share the steps taken by people with healthier lifespans.

The Blue Zones Food Guidelines are summarized as follows:

1. "95-100 plant-based foods"
2. "Go wholly whole" (reduce intake of processed foods)
3. "Daily dose of beans" (one or two servings of beans, chickpeas, lentils, or split peas)
4. "Drink mostly water"
5. "Snack on nuts"
6. "Go easy on fish"
7. "Eliminate eggs"
8. "Slash sugar"
9. "Reduce diary"
10. "Retreat from meat"

In a nutshell, this is excellent advice. My book will revisit some of these dietary recommendations.

Dan Buettner, in his book The Blue Zones: Secrets for Living Longer, interviewed Dr. Gary Frazier, the principal investigator of Adventist Health Studies in Loma Linda, California, one of the Blue Zones. Frazier has been researching thousands of Adventists for decades. "Clearly, a plant-based diet is the way to go," he said.

His second study, involving more than 96,000 participants since 2002, confirmed that strict vegetarian Adventists can expect to live longer than other Americans, with significantly fewer chronic diseases and cancers. In particular, the researchers calculated that vegetarian diets reduced the risk of developing type 2 diabetes by 50 percent and coronary heart disease by 60 percent. In contrast, Adventists who regularly eat meat have a 46 percent higher rate of premature death than those who get their proteins from nuts, seeds, and legumes. Frazier and his team also discovered an alarming connection between milk consumption and two types of cancer. Men who consume roughly 1 and 3/4 cups of milk per day face a 25 percent greater chance of developing prostate cancer. Women who drink as little as 1/4 cup of milk face 30 percent of developing breast cancer. One possible reason is the presence of cow hormones in milk from pregnant cows. To live longer and healthier, Frazier recommends:

1. Eat a vegetarian diet.
2. Get regular exercise.
3. Don't smoke.
4. Maintain a healthy body weight.
5. Snack on nuts.

Participants who followed these five habits experienced a ten-year boost in life expectancy. They not only lived longer but also lived better.

Adventists are more disciplined and resist the temptations of junk food more effectively than people in other Blue Zones, such as Okinawa and Nicoya in Costa Rica, where traditional lifestyles are disappearing.

Research studies show that high levels of IGF-1(Insulin-like Growth Factor) increase the risks of cancer, osteoarthritis, heart disease, and many other degenerative diseases related to aging. High protein diets raise IGF-1 levels. Eating bacon and eggs increases levels of IGF-1 and contributes to cancer cell growth. Dr. Dean Ornish and his colleagues were able to reverse the progression of early-stage, non-aggressive prostate cancer without chemotherapy, surgery, and radiation through a plant-based diet and a lifestyle program. It seems animal protein diets promote the development of cancer, while a plant-based diet appears to suppress it by switching off the expression of cancer growth genes at the genetic level. Suppose you consume large amounts of dairy after a prostate cancer diagnosis. In that case, you may suffer a 76 percent higher risk of death overall, and a 141 percent increased risk of dying specifically from cancer. The reduction of IGF-1 explains why vegans have lower rates of cancer. (Greger 77). Many magazines and books recommend a higher protein intake for people over 60. However, this advice can be risky if the protein is primarily animal-based. Switching to a plant-based diet to lower the levels of IGF-1 and prevent cancer development is a better option.

My wife and I have followed these recommendations for decades, even before the Blue Zone organization outlined them. Like the people in the Blue Zones, we realized decades ago that a plant-based system makes sense. My prescription, in fact, is a recommendation for a healthy lifestyle, summarized in the acronym DRESS-SS, which stands for diet, rest, exercise, sleep, stress management, sexuality and spirituality. Diet of this acronym, is the focus of this book.

Our Diet

We eliminated meat more than twenty years ago. We eat primarily wild salmon once a week. We reduced chicken to once a month. Chicken contains high levels of saturated fats and salt to increase their weight and raise their price, making it less healthy than promoted. We don't eat eggs or egg substitutes, as they contain saturated fats and are rich in methionine, an amino acid that shortens health and lifespan. We avoid farm-raised fish, including farm-raised salmon, due to their high content of harmful saturated fatty acids, methionine, and BCAAs. Most fish nowadays are contaminated with heavy metals like mercury. Farm-raised fish fed with corn, soy, and other grains, which fish cannot process, lead to higher levels of Arachidonic Acid (ARA) and harmful saturated fats. Almost all processed meats, such as bacon, baloney, sausages, hot dogs, hamburgers, and fried chicken, are responsible for the majority of heart attacks and strokes. These foods, prepared in fast-food restaurants, contain harmful oils rich in fats, palmitic oil, and particularly trans fats due to overheating. One of the worst foods is French fries.

We eat vegetables such as broccoli, spinach, kale salads, coleslaw, potato salads, sweet potatoes, celery, tomatoes, avocados, pickles, squash, cucumbers, carrots, onions, and garlic almost daily. These plant foods are rich in flavonoids like quercetin, which reduce inflammation and offer many other benefits to reduce degenerative diseases. We eat legumes like lentils, beans, and chickpeas once weekly as they are rich in antioxidants. We use olive oil, balsamic vinegar, and avocado oil, including for cooking. In the morning, we prepare smoothies by blending vegetables for fiber with fruits and almond milk. We add plant-based powder, glutamine, mushroom powder, omega-3, vitamin C, beet powder, moringa powder, and collagen powder to the smoothies. Our favorite fruits for the smoothies are strawberries or blueberries because they are rich in antioxidants. Sometimes, we prepare our smoothies with cold-pressed vegetable and fruit juice blends from manufacturers like Evolution Fresh and Suja Life. You can find them in many organic supermarkets. We also regularly eat fruits like blueberries, oranges, apples, strawberries, pineapple, watermelon, plums, and mangoes and in small amounts to maintain a low glycemic index.

We don't consume any dairy products. Cheese and milk are rich in saturated fats. We don't eat eggs anymore. We used to eat one or two eggs a week but eliminated them some time ago because of the high content of saturated fats, not cholesterol.

We don't use milk or eat cheese for many reasons. Prostate cancer is more prevalent in men who consume dairy, and due to cow estrogens in milk, women are more susceptible to breast and ovarian cancer. Diary is not a healthy food for adults and is responsible for many chronic inflammatory illnesses.

We eat whole grain bread, no more than two slices a day, and regularly consume walnuts, pistachios, macadamia nuts, and sesame seeds. In the evening, we prepare a turmeric-ashwagandha smoothie to help ensure a good night's sleep.

We adopted intermittent fasting more than twenty years ago. Our breakfast is around 10 to 11 a.m., and our last meal is about 5 to 6 p.m. We fast for at least 16 hours a day. Intermittent fasting helps keep our weight in check and raises our AMPK. Our BMI is under 25.

We don't drink alcohol, although we occasionally have a glass of wine. Clara, my wife, suffers from severe migraines when she consumes red wine. We don't use any sugars, syrups, honey or sweeteners., though we sometimes use stevia as a sweetener. Daily, we drink water with our meals and green tea or matcha, which is also rich in EGCG and antioxidants. Our diet is vegan, with the exception of salmon as a protein source. Some might say it is a vegetarian diet, except we don't eat dairy, pasta, or eggs. We don't count calories or restrict ourselves from eating any foods as long as they are plant-based. We avoid anything fried or containing harmful hydrogenated vegetable oils or animal fats. We believe that our diet prevents chronic inflammation, cardiovascular disease, strokes, degenerative diseases, autoimmune diseases, and decline of cognitive function. Our bodies look decades younger than our chronological age. Clara, my wife, looks twenty to thirty years younger than women of her chronological age. We feel full of energy, maintain an active social life, and read two or three books weekly. We also write books and articles and are avid ballroom dancers. We go to the gym twice a week and sleep from eight to nine hours at night. We don't experience significant stress and enjoy talking with friends and family.

Because of our wellness lifestyle, we decided to write books to help people live healthier lifestyles, prolong their longevity and love for life. Maintaining optimal weight is a bonus with this diet and lifestyle, but our focus is on weight loss, good health, avoiding degenerative diseases, and achieving healthier longevity. A plant-based diet is the foundation for achieving these goals. If you adopt this lifestyle, you could see the results within four weeks. Testing your lipid levels, thyroid levels, insulin levels, blood sugar, A1C, and inflammatory markers before you start is recommended to better assess your progress, but it is optional. You should educate yourself and become aware of the advances in nutritional science. We know more about nutrition and biological processes today than our ancestors did during Paleolithic times and even a hundred years ago. People in the Blue Zones live longer primarily because their diets are plant-based. However, they lack refrigeration and access to the variety of fresh fruits and vegetables we enjoy today. They also avoid processed foods and fast food restaurants that destroy the health of their customers every day.

What Influence Does Our Diet Have on Our Epigenome and DNA?

Some scientists estimate that about 25% of the risk of death is due to genetics, while the remaining 75% is influenced by diet, and other factors that determine our health and lifespan, says Luigi Fontana, a physician and codirector of the longevity research program at Washington University in St. Louis (quoted in Heid and O'Connor 2015).

In my opinion and based on my professional experience, diet plays a far more remarkable and significant role. Our diet influences our epigenome, which turns our genome and genetic code on and off.

The epigenome is a group of proteins or chemicals that operates above the DNA, activating genes through chemical reactions, such as adding or subtracting methyl radicals from foods.

One way diet affects the genes is through methylation.

What is DNA Methylation?

Food is a chemical that powerfully influences all chemical reactions in our biochemical system, including DNA methylation. DNA methylation can lower the chance of developing many hereditary diseases in the family. We can also control the expression of our genes by eating foods that turn on or off our DNA methylation. Methyl groups, which are chemical radicals found in many foods, help regulate DNA methylation. This communication occurs through the epigenome, like a music band director guiding the DNA on which gene to turn on or off.

Many of my wife's family members have type 2 diabetes, including one of our children. My wife is the only one without diabetes. She certainly has a genetic predisposition to diabetes, but with her diet low in sugars and carbohydrates, she has been able to suppress the expression of the diabetic gene. However, she remains vigilant. Any excess may at any time turn the diabetic gene on, and she could face the same challenges as the rest of her family is now. You can do the same, but suppressing the expression of the gene requires a great deal of discipline and a strict diet low in sugars and carbohydrates. A diet of less than 15 g of sugars or carbohydrates helps to keep the genes turned off.

Many foods are rich in methyl donors and influence many genes through DNA methylation. Other foods, called adaptogens, provide the molecules needed to regulate DNA methylation.

A lifestyle of wellness helps to foster healthy DNA methylation. These practices may include diet, rest, exercise, sleep, and stress management, all integral to my DRESS prescription.

In addition to diet, supplements rich in methyl groups can help either inhibit or promote gene expression. However, excessive methyl groups or hypermethylation can also be detrimental. Folate is a methyl donor vital for embryo development and cell regeneration. But, excessive folate in adults could lead to the development of cancer. The same may apply to B12 vitamins. If your folate and B12 levels are normal, there is no need for supplementation with these nutrients. Other influential methyl donors are Sam-e (S-adenosylmethionine), choline, betaine, zinc, magnesium, potassium, B vitamins (riboflavin, niacin, pyridoxine), amino acids, and omega3 fatty acids rich in DHA.

Since there are more than 20 million DNA methylation sites in each body cell, a deficiency of these nutrients will lead to an imbalanced DNA methylation system for the cells, which could have consequences for overall health. Many illnesses may stem from a DNA methylation deficit that leads to improper genetic expression or lack of expression.

DNA adaptogens are found in foods rich in flavonoids, such as polyphenols in green vegetables and fruits. Foods high in these flavonoids include turmeric (from the curcumin family), green tea, matcha (rich in EGCG), rosmarinic acid (from rosemary), quercetin, lycopene (found in tomatoes), sulforaphane (in cruciferous vegetables), and Vitamins A, C, and D3. These nutrients help regulate DNA methylation by adding or subtracting methyl groups for proper gene expression.

Why Do Many Diets Fail?

This information about DNA methylation is essential for understanding a healthy lifestyle. Most people are unaware of these critical biological reactions at the cellular level, which is why many diets and treatments fail. Most physicians don't fully understand many of these deficiencies or excesses of different nutrients and their consequences. These failures happen because most physicians don't receive nutritional training to know how to correct an illness or prevent deficiencies at the cellular level responsible for many degenerative diseases, diabetes, and cancer through proper dietary recommendations.

The Dietary Guidelines for Americans provide recommendations based on eating patterns. I will provide more information about the guidelines later in this chapter. I want to make clear that these Standard American Guidelines (SAD), although scientific, change every five years. They promote animal foods like meat, eggs, dairy, poultry, and fish, which are relatively low in minerals, vitamins, and plant-based foods and allow too many sugars and saturated fats. I am particularly concerned about the recommendations for fruit juices, sugar, and animal fats. The SAD contains only about two percent of calories from vegetables, which are some of the healthiest foods for preventing cardiovascular and degenerative diseases. Government guidelines should place stricter limits on sugar, saturated animal fats, and meats while emphasizing plant-based foods, more minerals and micronutrients.

When Should We Start to Get the Proper Nutrients?

Nutritional deficiencies can start as early as in utero. A mother deficient in folic acid will create a deficit in the fetus that can prevent the fetus from developing a healthy nervous system. Many children born with spine defects or brain problems, such as spina bifida, experienced folic acid deficiency during pregnancy. Women must be aware of these deficiencies to protect their children since they limit their likelihood of enjoying good health and a long life. Once a woman gets pregnant, she must educate herself about the potential effects of nutritional deficiencies, drugs, or behaviors that may affect her unborn child. Failing to do this could cause a heartache that will last a lifetime for both the mother and the innocent child.

Once we are born, mother's milk is an excellent food full of essential nutrients and protective antibodies that defend the child against various illnesses. As children grow and develop, they need more nutrients to help their bodies grow healthier. Mother's milk may be insufficient to feed a rapidly growing child. A nourishing formula or milk and additional foods should become part of an infant's diet to prevent nutritional deficiencies.

A well-balanced diet is essential for excellent development, helping to avoid defects and illnesses. One of the most catastrophic effects on the younger generation is the development of obesity. Parents play a significant role in the development of obesity in a child. Too much food leads to obesity, insulin resistance, and type 2 diabetes. A diet rich in carbohydrates and saturated fats may lead to permanent problems, becoming more apparent and profound as the child enters adulthood. Children's education about healthy foods and plant-based diets should be a priority at both home and school. Children must be responsible and learn to care for their bodies as the most precious possession and the source of ultimate happiness.

Who Are We?

We inherited from our ancestors the most magnificent gift ever created. Our bodies are the most advanced biochemical laboratories ever designed for survival on Earth. Unfortunately, the most advanced biochemical laboratories we own came without a clear and specific owner's manual. Our rudimentary operation manual came from our parents, who probably didn't know much about the body's capacities and cellular functions. Understanding how this sophisticated biochemical lab operates is essential to prevent illness and cure deficiencies for a healthier lifestyle before populating other planets.

From early childhood, it is crucial to understand our body's structure and how this remarkable lab processes all the chemicals we eat (as foods are essentially chemicals) and how they become living tissues and organs or how these chemicals interact to defend our bodies against our enemies by developing a defense system, make hormones, neurotransmitters and more products for a healthy existence and longevity. The crown jewel of such processes is our intelligence, which allows us to transform our environment and ensure the survival and preservation of consciousness in the universe. We have been fortunate to have survived on this hostile planet, yet we are still far away from learning more about who we are and what we are capable of achieving. One of the greatest shortcomings of modern medicine is the lack of training in medical schools regarding nutrition and how food and good nutrients can prevent or even cure many illnesses. Physicians have become too dependent on drug manufacturers to find cures, overlooking the power of healthy diets. Our ancestors survived without modern medications, as do most animals and plants. A diet rich in polyphenols and antioxidants, which counteracts the damaging effects of free radicals, should be a way to approach how to prevent damage to our DNA and organs. Healthy nutrients help to stop the development of plaques, cardiovascular diseases, degenerative diseases, cognitive decline, autoimmune disorders, cancer, and chronic inflammation. All these conditions are preventable. You can reach old age without any of these degenerative diseases, including cancer. A well-balanced diet free of saturated fats, toxic substances, excessive sugars or carbs, and the right amounts of essential amino acids, good fatty acids, minerals, and vitamins from birth would lead to healthier longevity free of the many illnesses we suffer today.

Hormones also contribute to healthy aging. IGF-1, or Insulin-like Growth Factor, is a powerful growth hormone structurally similar to insulin. Centenarians tend to have lower levels of this hormone. Animal models with lower levels of IGF-1 tend to live longer. Many researchers have been looking at the IGf-1 levels of the offspring and descendants of centenarians and have found that they share lower levels of this hormone. People with lower levels of IGF-1 enjoy better health and longevity. People born with the gene that produces lower hormone levels have an advantage. Those with higher levels should find ways to lower or decrease their levels as they age. We may consider a sign of more extended longevity to have low levels of IGF-1.

What Is Our Future?

Parents, governments, and schools must teach children to understand and care for this magnificent and advanced chemical laboratory, our body. In the same way, schools emphasize computer learning, they should underline with better education the workings of this extraordinary biochemical lab that makes us aware of what we do, who we are, and why we go to school to learn and transform the world around us. Children should know more about cell biology, genetics, the role of food, the metabolism of sugar intake and dangers, and how nutrients create new tissues and muscle mass and improve overall health. They should learn more about the structure of our immune system for our defense against many enemies and how to protect it and enhance it with a healthy lifestyle. I advocate for private schools dedicated to teaching these subjects. Suppose we are planning to go to other planets; this advanced education will be essential for future generations' survival, healthier lifestyles, and extended longevity. We are only beginning to scratch the surface of understanding how food and particular plant-based diets are essential for survival. We are growing in knowledge about how nutrients interact to improve our body functions.

The development of AI and quantum computing will further advance our understanding of chemical interactions and how our cells respond to any injury, repair tissues, or create new organs. We could follow chemical reactions and cellular functions in real-time. Medicine will be different decades from now. Our descendants will look back to our time as just another period of our primitive and outdated thinking, as we see today's primitives living in the Amazon jungle. The future promises brighter days and remarkable discoveries with a greater understanding of who we are, our purpose, and our destiny. It wouldn't be surprising if, in the millennia to come, we may reach a higher level of intelligence and powerful bodies capable of standing the rigors of our environment. The idea of becoming a superhuman or god-like figure is not far-fetched.

The Adverse Effects of a Poor diet

Obesity

The primary culprit of obesity is the consumption of and addiction to refined sugar. Parents should avoid giving sugary drinks like sodas or juices to their children. The amount of refined sugar in a soda is equivalent to ten teaspoons. Giving a can of soda full of sugar to a child or an adult is like giving them a slow poison, which eventually leads to obesity, diabetes, metabolic syndrome, and other complications, including damage to the nuclear DNA. Excessive sugar consumption generates excessive amounts of free radicals, which will damage the DNA and mitochondria. I advise any excellent parent to avoid sugary drinks as much as possible for anyone in your family. My advice also includes fruit juices containing excessive sugars like fructose and syrups. Avoid them like a plague. People wonder why juices are harmful since they come from fruits.

The reality is that manufacturers add sugars, even though fruits already contain complex sugars, which take longer to absorb. They make these additions to make juices more palatable. I recommend buying fresh orange juice using natural fruit with less than 50 percent sugar. Alternatively, squeezing oranges or blending an apple, strawberries, and bananas to make fresh juice and smoothies is a healthier choice.

Note: The American Academy of Pediatrics recommends against giving fruit juices to children under one year of age since this contributes to the development of obesity.

Eating fruit in moderation is fine, but you should be aware of the glycemic index. Many fruits have a higher content of glucose and fructose content.

Fructose, in particular is problematic for the liver to metabolize and tends to be stored as fat. Sugars raise the levels of insulin and contribute to obesity. A regular-sized banana contains the equivalent of ten teaspoons of sugar. If you are overweight, pay attention to the consumption of fruits. Cut the fruit in half to lower the sugar content. Many scientific studies suggest that eating fruits and vegetables makes people happier and healthier (Longo 2018; Murray 2017). If you are trying to lose weight, consuming excessive amounts of fruits may cause you to gain weight. A banana has a high glycemic index and contains complex sugars that take longer to absorb. If you are on a diet, eating two bananas a day is equal to one can of soda a day. That is why people who are trying to lose weight do not lose weight. They feel they are eating the right foods rich in vegetables and fruits but see no change. Fruits provide good nutrients and complex carbohydrates, minerals, vitamins, flavonoids like quercetin, and antioxidants for more energy. These complex carbohydrates take longer to digest and are difficult to absorb as fast as refined sugars. However, too many fruits with a high glycemic index will make you gain weight. One orange or apple provides enough vitamins and nutrients for a day.

The excessive daily consumption of carbohydrates, whether from refined sugars, flour, bread, alcohol, wine, or syrups, is another contributing factor to obesity, diabetes, and metabolic syndrome. Limit your intake of carbohydrates; one or two slices of whole grain bread are sufficient with a meal, rather than a half loaf of white bread. Just as with fruits, when eating carbohydrates, the key is moderation. To delay the absorption of these complex carbohydrates, I recommend adding fiber. You may eat a carrot or blend carrots and vegetables in a blender to prepare your smoothies. Research and many reports in the literature emphasize plant-based diets as the healthiest diets to maintain good health and extended longevity. I modified the diet recommendations listed in my first book. My recommendation is to eliminate meats, most animal foods, and animal fats since they are rich in saturated fats. Plants contain sufficient protein to build muscle and new tissues. You must observe the animals and see if they survive on plant food alone. Elephants, buffaloes, cattle, and horses consume only vegetables. For billions of years, most animals survived on plant-based foods as the only source of nutrients. Animals don't refine sugars or eat junk food as humans do. Adding greens to our diet is a way to live healthy lives and grow stronger. Mediterranean diets are acceptable, except for consuming too much pasta, bread, eggs, poultry, and carbohydrates. I lean toward recommending a vegan or modified vegetarian diet, free of saturated fats, as the baseline for healthy living.

Is a plant-based diet the ultimate solution for better health?

Table 1. Foods rich in antioxidants

Rank	Food	Size	Total antioxidant capacity per serving size
1	Small red bean (dried)	half cup	13,727
2	Wild blueberry	1 cup	13,427
3	Red kidney bean (dried)	half cup	13,259
4	Pinto bean	half cup	11,864
5	Blueberry (cultivated)	1 cup	9,019
6	Cranberry	1 cup (whole)	8,983
7	Artichoke (cooked)	1 cup (hearts)	7,904
8	Blackberry	1 cup	7,701
9	Prune	half cup	7,291
10	Raspberry	1 cup	6,058
11	Strawberry	1 cup	5,938
12	Red Delicious apple	1 whole	5,900
13	Granny Smith apple	1 whole	5,381
14	Pecan	1 ounce	5,095
15	Sweet cherry	1 cup	4,873
16	Black plum	1 whole	4,844
17	Russet potato (cooked)	1 whole	4,649
18	Black bean (dried)	half cup	4,181
19	Plum	1 whole	4,118
20	Gala apple	1 whole	3,903

Public information from USDA. Reviewed by Charlotte E Grayson Mathis MD. 2005 for WebMD.

Diets to be healthier and lose weight

Plant-based foods are the most beneficial foods for a healthy lifestyle and longevity. A healthy diet should include wild fish and nuts. I no longer recommend chicken or turkey because of the high-fat content. Chicken contains saturated fats and salt added during its processing. Most greens are healthful and are rich in vitamins, antioxidants, fiber, and protein. Adding greens to any diet is a key step to living a healthier life and increasing vitality. Eating veggies every day is a healthy practice. My recommendation is to follow a plant-based diet rich in antioxidants as a means of controlling weight and improving health. Consuming less than 15 g of carbohydrates per day and caloric restriction help keep your AMPK activated and decrease your craving for more food. An intermittent fasting diet also helps to keep your weight in check. Several veggies a day should be part of a good diet. Unfortunately, most children reject vegetables in their diets. Why? Parents fail to introduce them very early in the child's development. They mistakenly believe that junk food rich in sugar is good for appeasing their children for good behaviors and using it as a reward. The practice of rewarding children with sugary drinks, ice cream, and fast food is a horrible mistake. Hamburgers, French fries, and fried foods low in fiber are some of the worst foods to feed a child. A diet associated with soda, ice cream, and pizza, hot dogs, cheese is rich in saturated fats and sugars that contribute to obesity, metabolic syndrome, nonalcoholic fatty liver, and coronary artery disease; it is not healthy and will lead to many health problems as the child grows up. Unfortunately, parents give these kinds of foods to their children. The same foods are prevalent in school cafeterias. When parents use junk food for their children as a reward, they send the wrong message and fail to help them develop good eating behaviors for a healthy, long life. Junk diets accelerate the development of illnesses predisposed by our genetic code, one of the most common being diabetes. Adding foods with excessive sugars to a diet is like fueling a fire. Children and adults with a predisposition to diabetes or heart disease should avoid junk foods. Good behaviors start with proper and responsible guidance from parents. Again, instant gratification with sugary drinks and foods for good deeds is detrimental. Awareness, education, and discipline are necessary for developing good behaviors. If parents fail to introduce good foods in infancy, their children will likely grow up eating harmful junk foods. The consequences will not be immediate but cumulative over many years. In my many years as a medical doctor, I have seen many men and women dying of heart disease very early in their lives. Unfortunately, obesity in children today is typical. Generally, these children can trace their obesity to the learned behaviors from their parents. Children should learn from their parents to appreciate which foods are healthy.

Greens, well-cooked or fresh, can be a delicious treat. Using them to prepare shakes or drinks combined with fruits is a way to introduce greens into a child's diet. I do not dispute the value of eating greens. Some people are concerned that veggies do not provide proteins. They are wrong. Greens can supply all the proteins necessary for all body functions, particularly those of a growing child. We need to look only at animals feeding from grass. Cattle develop into big and powerful animals that give us milk and meat to feed our bodies. They do not consume steaks, fish, sugar, sugary drinks, or fatty foods. They are essentially grass eaters that can fully develop without eating the foods we consume daily. Most greens contain essential amino acids, minerals, fiber, antioxidants, carotenoids, flavonoids, and a full spectrum of enzymes and minerals required for a healthy life. The goal is to develop a behavior for a diet that combines vegetables and fruits every day of our lives. Veggies are alkaline and these help combat acidosis. An alkaline diet helps to digest foods, improve metabolism, and increase energy. Blending veggies and fruits in a blender is a way to make shakes and juices that children and adults enjoy. I frequently recommend these smoothies to my patients who are debilitated by illness or who want to lose weight. Look for some of my favorite smoothies made of fruits and veggies in Appendix A. If you prefer, rather than preparing vegetable-based dishes or eating whole fruits and vegetables, you can substitute fruit and vegetable smoothies to help you ingest the recommended daily quota of natural fruit and vegetables.

You can make smoothies from many different kinds of fruits and vegetables. Blending fruits and vegetables is a way to get several servings of fruits and vegetables each day. Examples of good fruits for powerful smoothies are apples, blueberries, strawberries, bananas, dried plums, cherry juice extract, grapes, or kiwi. Remember that avocado is an excellent fruit with good polyunsaturated fats. Examples of good vegetables to add are carrots, spinach, kale, celery, broccoli, squash, cucumbers, quinoa, and beets. Surprisingly, none of these vegetables detract from the taste and flavors.

Commercial smoothies are not suitable for you as these smoothies contain too much sugar. A better smoothie is when fresh fruits and vegetables are available at home as they are rich in antioxidants that help prevent DNA damage. Packaged frozen fruits are acceptable since they can be stored in the freezer to avoid damage to the fruits. You can prepare your own or find them at your local grocery store, ready to be placed in the blender. Orange juice squeezed from the fruit is the best. A smoothie should contain at least 3 grams of fiber. Add flax seed, squash, or celery for fiber. Fiber slows down sugar absorption, leading to weight gain and more abdominal fat. A smoothie should contain protein to be nutritious.

You can add plant-based protein powder to provide polyphenols, antioxidants, and all amino acids necessary for all body functions or to increase muscle mass. I start my mornings with my "morning essentials," which combine omega-3 and fresh orange juice smoothies to provide two essential nutrients our bodies do not produce on their own—omega-3 fatty acids and vitamin C.

Need another reason to eat your greens? Recent research shows that people who follow a plant-based diet are less likely to have specific "bad" bacteria in their gut that increase the risk for diabetes and heart disease.

A metagenomic study of the gut microbes from more than 1,000 individuals found a statistically significant overlap between the gut microbiome and a healthy diet and positive markers for cardiovascular health, including a lower likelihood of diabetes and obesity. Researchers identified which study participants ate primarily plant-based diets based on their self-reported food diaries. A plant-based diet promotes a healthy microbiome.

Both Vegetarians and Vegans Are at a Decreased Risk for Obesity and Heart-Related Diseases

A vegetarian diet excludes animal meat but allows for dairy intake. In contrast, those following a vegan diet avoid all animal products. Both vegetarians and vegans are at a decreased risk of obesity and many heart-related diseases; vegans specifically are less likely to have unhealthy cholesterol levels—which makes sense since saturated animal fats can contribute to high cholesterol.

While a plant-based diet does not necessarily limit simple sugars that can contribute to diabetes, a vegetarian diet may still benefit people with diabetes due to its emphasis on heart-healthy fruits and vegetables.

Whether you eat a plant-based diet, fish or limited amounts of meat, you can achieve a healthy balance in your microbiome through probiotic intake and regular intake of nutritious foods, including fermented foods like kimchi, miso, and sauerkraut—all of which are commonly found in vegetarian dishes.

A study published in the March 2021 issue of *Nature Medicine* connecting eating vegetarian diets to heart health is not the only recent report showing the health benefits of a vegetarian diet. A UK study of more than 177.000 British adults showed reduced heart disease and cancer risk.

In Appendix A, I provide recipes for smoothies and healthy beverages to start your day, along with the best healthy veggie-fruit smoothies for you and your family. These smoothies could be the basis for a healthy diet and help with weight loss and reduction of unwanted fat. If you have no time in the morning, you can prepare them the night before.

Children will enjoy these smoothies and learn to add veggies and fruits to their diets.

In Appendix A, I also describe some of my favorite desserts. My coconut blueberry yogurt delight is rich in antioxidants and probiotics. Obesity is an epidemic spreading across America.

It is associated with numerous health problems and complications, such as hypertension, diabetes, atherosclerosis, heart disease, metabolic syndrome, low back pain, arthritis, degeneration of the joints, premature aging, and loss of productivity. People who are obese usually develop insulin resistance and diabetes, leading to a metabolic syndrome. Recent research (Taubes 2016, 258–62) indicates that people with insulin resistance and high levels of insulin and insulin-like growth factor are more likely to develop cancer. These changes happen because the cells affected begin to modify how they use sugar for energy through aerobic glycolysis. During this process, insulin and insulin-like growth factor (IGF) allow the cells to utilize large amounts of sugar as an energy source for rapid proliferation. During this production of large amounts of energy, the cells release free radicals, which cause damage to the mitochondria and the nuclear DNA, leading to mutations and the development of cancer. This process suggests that there is a cause-and-effect relationship between elevated sugar levels and the development of cancer (Murray 2017, 68–71).

A carbohydrate-rich diet not only causes damage at the cellular and organ level but also at the societal level, affecting the individual, the family, personal finances, and the national economy.

The associated medical care costs are staggering. The cost associated with the loss of productivity and healthcare adds up to trillions of dollars.

It is hard to believe that all these problems stem from poor eating habits, lack of proper education, and destructive behaviors from childhood. These costs and health problems are tragedies that parents, teachers, and educators can prevent at home and school through awareness, education, and discipline.

We all have a life and a body to protect, and learning to live healthily from childhood is essential. We can correct unhealthy behaviors and lifestyles through education at home and school. We must not continue to ignore the obesity epidemic that is killing people prematurely and affecting their health, longevity, finances, the cost of healthcare, and the pursuit of happiness.

How Can Free Radicals Cause Cancer?

Diets rich in carbohydrates create an unhealthy environment where free radicals constantly bombard the cells. These free radicals, which are unstable atoms like hydrogen or byproducts of glucose metabolism in addition to ATP, CO_2, and water, can damage cellular structures. CO_2 leaves the cell, proceeds to the vein system, and then to the lungs, where it leaves as CO_2. Water leaves through the kidneys. Billions of cells are constantly working to keep this process going and to maintain healthy energy levels. This process occurs in the mitochondria, which act as a factory or power plant. For example, in a power plant, the raw materials are carbohydrates. Once the carbs enter the membrane, they pass into a conveyor belt called Kreb's cycle. The free radicals create a polluted environment that requires fast removal.

Since these chemicals lack one electron, they are highly unstable. They search for additional electrons and try to steal them from nearby proteins or compounds. One of the proteins is the DNA. Removing one electron from one amino acid in the DNA sequences can change the structure and function of the DNA. This defective DNA, in effect, mutates, providing different information to subsequent cells. If the mutation activates the oncogenic genes, the final result is a cancerous cell. Cancer cells keep growing at a fast rate without control. It seems they want to become independent from the self and develop at their own pace without regard for the whole. Since they require a great deal of energy, they utilize large amounts of ATP, producing exponential quantities of free radicals and damaging more cells nearby during the process.

Why Can't People Lose Weight Despite a Low-Carb Diet?

When a person has diabetes, there is too much sugar outside the cell waiting to pass through the cell membrane, but the door is closed. Insulin stops doing its job because most of the receptors for insulin in the membrane are full. There is no place or seat for the extra insulin outside the cell, resulting in an accumulation of glucose reflected by elevated blood sugar levels. This dysfunction is called Insulin resistance. This polluted environment worsens when one consumes carbohydrates and refined sugars daily and at night. No wonder people with these types of diets eventually become sick, develop type 2 diabetes, and become obese. The good news is that the diabetic can reverse this dreadful situation and environment. Reducing and substantially eliminating carbs from diets helps clean up the pollution and reduce the oxidative process, taxing the mitochondria and the cells' functions. People will lose weight with less sugar or carbs, allowing the cells to utilize their fat deposits as energy sources. This fact is evident in those who have had gastric bypasses and see their blood sugar levels returning to normal. Also, insulin or hypoglycemic medications are no longer required.

Can We Improve Our Quality of Life with a Fasting Ketogenic Diet?

In my practice, I sometimes recommend a "fast-keto diet" for people who struggle to lose weight. To lose weight on this diet, a person should stop eating after 6: 00 p.m. and fast until 10.00 a.m. the following day to have a minimum of sixteen hours of fasting. This period allows the body to switch from carbohydrates as a fuel to fat and ketones. Exercising helps to remove more fat. Energy will come from ketones first and fat later from fat stored, not from a fat diet. Fat has nine calories per gram, so consuming too much fat from food can limit the release of stored fat from deposits around your belly. The liver releases the ketones into the blood. All cells can take ketones from the blood and reconvert them into acetyl-CoA, which can then be used in the mitochondria to fuel their citric acid cycles. Stored fatty acids are broken down to acetyl-CoA through beta-oxidation inside the mitochondria, reverting into sugar as an energy source by the cells. The burning of excess fat is the mechanism behind hibernation. Large animals, like bears, prepare for winter by accumulating fat. When winter comes and food is limited, they use stored fat to survive. They don't consume more fat and lose weight. Such a mechanism is still present in humans. The problem is that food is plentiful, and some people continue to eat without control as if preparing for hibernation. If a person tries to lose weight by fasting for a few more hours, the body will use fat stored in the liver and muscles first; then, the body is in a state of nutritional ketosis. Ketones become the energy source, and the body prepares to burn the fat stored in the belly. You can test if you are in nutritional ketosis using a dipstick to check the urine for ketone bodies. You can find this dipstick at any pharmacy. It typically take two or three days to achieve nutritional ketosis.

When cells use ketones for fuel, the production of free radicals decreases at the mitochondria, preventing mitochondrial and DNA damage. Several studies suggest that reducing sugar and carbohydrates for fats only as fuel decreases the amount of sugar in cancer cells that depend on this fuel source. Cancer cells grow very fast and require significant amounts of carbohydrates to develop. Decreasing the number of sugars slows or stops the development of cancer cells.

Ketones reduce inflammation by decreasing pro-inflammatory cytokines. In addition, ketosis inhibits the mTOR pathway, improving health span and lifespan.

A healthier diet incorporates intermittent fasting, low carbs diet, and use ketones as an additional energy source. I recommend this fast-keto diet because it reduces the production of damaging free radicals and helps you keep your weight down.

In her book about ketogenic diets, nutritionist Miriam Kalamian, relates how her son, who had brain cancer, improved significantly with a ketogenic diet. He lived six more years after his doctors had nothing else to offer. Her story is very compelling and makes sense as a way to slow down cancer cells from developing.

Personally, as a clinician, if you have cancer or any of your loved ones have cancer, I recommend reducing carbs to no more than 15 g a day to allow nutritional ketosis and fat burning.

Sugar is addictive.

Sugar is addictive, which is why many people gain weight or cannot lose it.

Sugar induces a pleasurable response in the brain's "reward center" in a similar way to nicotine, heroin, cocaine, and alcohol. It also stimulates the release of dopamine, which provides a pleasant reaction identical to the potent effects of other addictive drugs. Like many addictions, when fewer dopamine receptors become available, the need for more sugar becomes more intense to maintain a pleasurable response.

Sugar causes the body to produce insulin to keep blood sugar within a normal range. Excessive amounts of sugar signal the cells that more sugar is available outside the cell membrane. However, the lack of sufficient insulin receptors creates insulin resistance, preventing sugar from being transported into the cells. The increased blood sugar and high levels of insulin trigger the production of more free radicals, which in turn damage the DNA and may lead to the development of cancer. The cells create more receptors to accept the sugar on the outside to accommodate the excess sugar, a situation seen in type 2 diabetes. The lack of insulin characterizes type 1 diabetes. In type 2 diabetes, the abnormal sugar metabolism creates a resistance to insulin at the cell level. In the brain, as is the case with narcotics, sugar stimulates the reward centers, leading to addiction. As insulin levels increase, leptin and growth hormone levels, which regulate energy and appetite, decrease. If the diet is rich in carbohydrates, leptin and growth hormone production eventually stops, leading to an uncontrollable appetite, weight gain, obesity, fatigue, and low energy. To fight these symptoms, a person has to stop consuming sugars to end the addiction and help the body return to an average balance and metabolic equilibrium. During this period, a person may experience symptoms of withdrawal the same way many people with an addiction to narcotics feel when they quit cold turkey. Once leptin and growth hormone levels rise, the appetite and a sensation of fullness come under control. A person addicted to sugar begins to feel better. The production of dopamine gradually decreases. The cravings for sugary drinks stop, food tastes better, sleep improves, thirst diminishes, and weight begins to drop.

At this point, clothes begin to feel loose as the body starts using fat as energy. The feedback mechanisms return because there is an internal balance when all chemistries and hormones in the sugar metabolism cycle are in equilibrium. When balance returns, a person on a diet begins to lose weight. Cells overwhelmed by excess sugar 24-7 create a feeling of tiredness and lack of energy. This feeling goes away as fat leaves from the deposits all over the body. Removing this excess fat is the first step to losing weight and eliminating the addiction to sugars. To start losing weight, you have to make a choice and a conscious decision to eat properly and maintain a healthy lifestyle. You will fail without a mental decision and determination to lose weight and live a healthier lifestyle.

However, don't get discouraged. Even if you have done your best to watch your diet and exercise but failed, there are still some ways to help you. The best approach is to have a physical examination and ask your doctor to do some lab tests to check your thyroid, insulin levels, blood sugar, HbA1c, lipid panel, and sex hormones as a baseline for monitoring your health and keep a record of your progress. A1C represents the average of three months of blood sugar. If you have been diligent about your diet and haven't lost weight over six months, you should consider a lap-band procedure or gastric bypass. In my experience, people who had these procedures lost significant weight and had minimal complications. It is essential to see a surgeon with expertise and successful outcomes. Many of my patients who had these procedures lost weight, had normal blood sugar levels, and did not need insulin or other hypoglycemic agents, and most importantly, they felt healthier and happier.

Are Drugs Like Ozempic Good for Losing Weight?

Ozempic and similar drugs are used to control blood sugar and are not for weight loss. They belong to a group of medicines known as Glucagon-like peptide-1(GLP-1) drugs. Some doctors are using this drug off-label for weight loss. The drug is through injection once a week. It works by mimicking incretin, a hormone that regulates the amount of insulin released into the blood after eating, lessening glucagon secretion by the stomach and slowing the movement of food through the stomach, causing a sensation of fullness and lowering appetite. Some people have lost weight and claim to feel better. However, there are complications. One of the problems is gastroparesis, which means the stomach is paralyzed or is not moving. Other side effects are diarrhea, nausea, constipation, high blood lipase, and amylase. It would be best to never try these medicines first without trying diet as recommended in this book.

How Does Caloric Restriction Help Us to Lose Weight?

Table 2. A low carb diet for a healthier life and to lose weight

Fruits per cup	Vegetables	Nuts and seeds	Beverages
Avocado	Asparagus	Almonds	Almond milk
Blackberries	Beets	Brazil nuts	Coconut milk
Berries 1/2 a cup	Broccoli	Cashews	Broth
Blueberries 1/2 a cup	Brussels Sprouts	Chia	Coffee decaf
Cranberries	Cabbage	Coconuts	Coffee unsweetened
Grapefruit	Carrots	Flaxseed seeds	Tea unsweetened
Lemon	Cauliflower	Flaxseed meal	Water
Lime	Celery	Hazelnuts	
Raspberries	Cucumber	Macadamia nuts	
Strawberries	Eggplant	Pecans	
Half an apple	Garlic	Pistachios	
Half an orange	Green beans	Pumpkin seeds	
Half a pear	Kale	Sunflower seeds	
Pineapple small slice	Mushrooms	Walnuts	
Watermelon small wedge or 1/2 cup diced	Okra		
	Onions		
	Peppers		
	Pumpkin		
	Salad greens		
	Spinach		
	Tomatoes		
	Zucchini		

Another way to lose weight is through caloric restriction. Fasting and a low-calorie diet stimulate the elevation of AMPK, which is a master energy sensor that helps to control the accumulation of fat. When there is not enough food, AMPK activity increases, and the body enters a period of stress, triggering the activity of AMPK to start a conservation period. AMPK (AMP-activated protein kinase) is an enzyme that detects the depletion of fuel in animals and plants. It acts as the gauge sensor in a car when we are running low on gas. When the sensor shows we are very low on gas, the cells utilize fat as an energy source from its deposits. In other words, we are like a hybrid car. The body switches from electric or gas to another kind of energy source. Burning fat by this mechanism affects weight loss as well as longevity. Calorie restriction and activated AMPK contribute to an extended lifespan. Animal studies show that the lifespan of worms and mice increases with AMPK activators. Supplements that elevate AMPK are available on the market and help create a feeling of starvation to activate fat burning from deposits.

Some foods impair AMPK. Saturated fats suppress AMPK.

Dr. Michael Greger, in his book *"How Not to Age,"* states all saturated fats, particularly palmitic acid.. This particular fat is present in meat and dairy fat. Saturated fats are responsible for metabolic diseases, cardiovascular disease, cancer, neurodegenerative diseases, and inflammation.

Saturated fats are toxic to the liver. Nonalcoholic fatty liver has become the leading cause of liver disease in the world. Many studies estimate that from 75 to 100 million people have this liver disease in the USA, or one in three Americans. The overaccumulation of fat in the liver is due to the overconsumption of calories. Sugar is one source, but saturated fat is even worse. Candy and sugars increase fat in the liver by 33%, but saturated fats, like the ones in meat, milk, and cheese, increase liver fat by 55%. Unsaturated fats like olive or avocado oil don't inhibit AMPK activation as saturated fats.

Foods that activate and boost AMPK include berberine (found in barberries), hibiscus tea, lemon verbena, and apple vinegar.

How Are Fatty Acids Oxidized to Provide Energy?

Fatty acids are converted into acetyl-CoA through beta-oxidation inside the mitochondria. Fatty acid oxidation starts on the outer mitochondrial membrane. The fatty acids, which, like carbohydrates, are relatively inert, must first be activated by conversion to an energy-rich fatty acid derivative of coenzyme A. The enzyme responsible for this activation is *acetyl*-CoA *synthetase.* For each molecule of fatty acid-activated, one molecule of coenzyme A and one molecule of adenosine triphosphate (ATP) are used, equaling a net utilization of the two high-energy bonds in one ATP molecule.

The fate of the acetyl-CoA obtained from fatty acid oxidation depends on an organism's needs. It may enter the citric acid cycle pathway and be oxidized to produce energy or a different pathway for the formation of water-soluble derivatives known as ketone bodies, or it may serve as the starting material for the synthesis of fatty acids. These ketone bodies lead to ketosis. Nutritional ketosis shouldn't be confused with diabetic ketoacidosis, which is a severe condition. This diet is essentially an intermittent fasting diet, not a starvation diet.

In starvation, diabetes mellitus, and other physiological conditions in which cells do not receive sufficient amounts of carbohydrates, the rate of ketone body formation in the liver increases further to a level much higher than can be used by other tissues. The excess ketone bodies accumulate in the blood and the urine, a condition referred to as *ketosis.* When the acetone in the blood reaches the lungs, its volatility causes a smell in the breath. The sweet smell of acetone, a characteristic of ketosis, is frequently noticed on the breath of severely diabetic patients.

Because two of the three kinds of ketone bodies are weak acids, their presence in the blood in excessive amounts overwhelms the blood buffers and causes a marked decrease in blood pH (to 6.9 from a standard value of 7.4). This decrease in pH leads to a severe condition known as ***acidosis.*** One effect of acidosis is a decrease in the ability of hemoglobin to transport oxygen in the blood. In moderate to severe acidosis, breathing becomes difficult and very painful. The body also loses fluids and becomes dehydrated as the kidneys attempt to eliminate the acids by removing large quantities of water. The lowered oxygen supply and dehydration lead to depression; even mild acidosis leads to lethargy, loss of appetite, and a general run-down. Without urgent treatment, a patient may die.

I want to caution people with diabetes to be careful to avoid entering ketoacidosis.

Are We Rusting and Oxidizing Continuously?

Yes. Oxidative stress is a bodily condition caused by low antioxidant levels, and it is an ongoing process. When you open an apple or an avocado, within a few hours, it turns dark due to oxidation. Similarly, our skin and body are under constant stress due to oxidation. Too much oxidative stress damages tissues and causes premature aging. We must fight oxidation with a diet rich in antioxidants.

There is an imbalance of reactive oxygen species (ROS), also known as free radicals and antioxidants, and your body experiences oxidative stress. This imbalance can play a role in certain illnesses and conditions like diabetes.

Oxidative stress can lead to cell and tissue breakdown and DNA damage. However, this imbalance may also have some benefits.

What to Know About Oxidative Stress?

While oxidative stress harms overall health, it can have some uses. Some research has shown that oxidative stress may affect specific diseases. Measuring oxidant and antioxidant levels in the body can help researchers understand how these levels impact particular diseases.

Oxidative stress has more harmful properties than helpful ones. It can break down cell tissue and cause mitochondrial and DNA damage. This damage can also result in inflammation, which can lead to diabetes or cancer in some cases.

Can Excessive Sugar Intake Cause Cancer?

Previously, in this chapter, we addressed this question regarding the damage done to the mitochondrial and nuclear DNA when a diet is rich in sugars or carbohydrates. In 1930, German physiologist Otto Warburg—a Nobel laureate—discovered that cancer cells use glucose as fuel, consuming and metabolizing the sugar at a far higher rate than normal cells. Recent research shows that cancer may be related to high sugar and insulin levels. In 2003, epidemiologists from the Centers for Disease Control (CDC), led by Eugenia Calle, published an analysis in The New England Journal of Medicine reporting that cancer mortality in the United States is associated with obesity and being overweight. Heavier individuals were more likely to die from cancer than their leaner counterparts. In 2004, the CDC did an analysis linking cancer to diabetes, particularly pancreatic, colorectal, liver, bladder, and breast cancers. The clue was the finding of cancer in individuals who were not obese but suffered metabolic syndrome and were insulin resistant. The research showed that people with higher levels of insulin and an insulin-like growth factor (IGF) had a greater likelihood of getting cancer.

In 2005, Scottish researchers reported that people with diabetes who took metformin, a drug used to lower insulin resistance, had significantly lower levels of insulin and a reduced risk of cancer when compared to other diabetics on other medications. These findings suggest that hyperglycemia, high insulin resistance, and an IGF presence are cancer promoters.

Further research demonstrated that cancer cells are addicted to insulin to survive. In cultures, cancer cells die if no insulin is available. Researchers at the National Cancer Institute found that breast cancer cells are susceptible to insulin because they have receptors sensitive to insulin, something lacking in healthy breast tissue. Tumor cells have three to four times more receptors sensitive to IGF.

Researchers like Lewis Cantley and Craig Thompson believe that cancer is as much a metabolic disease as a "proliferative" disease (quoted in Taubes 2016). Genetic mutations are responsible for these changes. Cancer, as a metabolic disease, uses insulin and IGF as promoters through various steps.

First, insulin and IGF elevate blood sugar and insulin resistance which causes cells to utilize a mechanism of aerobic glycolysis, similar to what bacteria use in oxygen-poor environments. Once the cancer cells make this conversion, they begin to burn enormous amounts of energy, using glucose as fuel, which allows them to reproduce exponentially. Thompson suggests that when the cells use large amounts of sugar, they generate large amounts of free radicals, damaging the DNA and causing mutations. This new kind of cell proliferates quickly using large amounts of energy. At about this time, the high insulin and IGF levels signal the cancer cells to keep growing.

Researchers are concerned that the high levels of sucrose and fructose in our foods raise insulin resistance. Fructose is lipogenic and deposited as fat since the liver can't metabolize it. Research studies demonstrate that a diet rich in sucrose and fructose causes fatty liver and weight gain. Removing these sugars from the diet helps individuals lose weight and fat from their livers.

You can take preventive steps to lower your risk of developing cancer by following these steps:

1. Reduce sugar intake to less than 5% of your daily calories.
2. Keep your BMI under 25.
3. Avoid sugars like sucrose and fructose. They make you gain weight because they are lipogenic.
4. Eating healthy. Include vegetables and whole grains in your diet to add fiber. Decrease your consumption of saturated fats. Use healthy plant oils like olive oil and avocado oil. Eat fruits with a low glycemic index and in small amounts.
5. Exercise every day, at least 20 minutes of vigorous exercise.
6. Avoid alcohol. Alcohol turns into acetaldehyde, which is carcinogenic.
7. Avoid smoking.
8. Avoid processed foods. Many contain carcinogens like nitrosamines.
9. Avoid meat and overcooked meats. They are associated with colorectal cancer.
10. Avoid dairy products. Milk and cheese are rich in saturated fats; they also contain sugars and cow estrogens that may cause breast cancer and prostate cancer.

Can Foods Cause Inflammation?

Yes. Some foods and substances in foods, like additives, insecticides, fungicides, heavy metals, and molds or mycotoxins, play a crucial role in developing chronic inflammation. Consuming saturated fat increases pro-inflammatory markers, particularly in diabetics and overweight people. However, this can affect anyone, regardless of genetic predisposition. Synthetic trans fats in hydrogenated oils increase inflammatory markers, specifically IL-6 TNF-alpha, in overweight individuals.

Overheated oils are used every day in fast-food chains and restaurants, are particularly harmful. These oils can damage your body, increase the risk of obesity, and damage your arteries. Unfortunately, many people are not aware of this fact, which contributes to millions of cases of cardiovascular disease, obesity, cancer, autoimmune disorders, and mental illness.

Consequently, we see an increase in inflammation-related diseases such as heart disease, atherosclerosis, heart attacks, obesity, diabetes, and cancer.

It becomes essential for your survival that you do more to prevent chronic inflammation and damage to your intestinal wall, arteries, and many organs by limiting the consumption of saturated fats and foods triggering an inflammatory response as much as possible.

Some people who eat excessive amounts of meat or fish develop gout, a disease that causes intense pain and inflammation of the joints.

People predisposed to an elevation of uric acid develop deposits of urate crystals in soft tissues and joints. The crystals may form in the kidneys with severe consequences. Meat is rich in purines, produces high uric acid levels when metabolized. Many foods trigger allergies or food sensitivities, leading to inflammation of the intestinal wall and chronic inflammation.

Diet Recommendations

What Is a Balanced Diet?

To have a balanced diet, we need proteins, healthy fats, carbohydrates, minerals, vitamins, and antioxidants in the appropriate amounts to keep the body healthy and prevent disease. A balanced diet varies depending on your body size, gender, age, and physical activity.

Despite its freshness and preparation, food may contain toxic substances like fungicides, insecticides, hormones, antibiotics, heavy metals, mold toxins, or mycotoxins that negatively affect our health. The problem is that these toxins are difficult to detect. Some are part of plants that use them to defend against insects and other animals. When these toxins enter the digestive system, they trigger an inflammatory response. Many illnesses and autoimmune disorders are related to chronic inflammation in the lining of the intestinal wall.

Allergies, and food sensitivities are responsible for many symptoms that are difficult to explain. Bloating, fatigue, brain fog, body aches, joint pain, and lack of optimal cognitive performance are symptoms of chronic inflammation. There are ways to find out which foods may be triggering these symptoms. It would help to ask your doctor to run one of these tests. If he does not know, you should look for a doctor specializing in functional or lifestyle medicine. A GI specialist could also help with the investigation. Removing the offending agent removes the symptoms and improves your health.

Some foods may trigger an autoimmune disease and could cause devastating damage. Examples are lupus, rheumatoid arthritis, inflammatory bowel syndrome or IBS, and many more. Most recently, there have been reports of patients with severe mental illness secondary to an autoimmune disorder. Schizophrenia, psychosis, and catatonic schizophrenia have been associated with antibodies in the receptors of nerve membranes in the brain interfering with the transmission of nerve impulses, causing an imbalance of neurotransmitters for optimal nerve function. Many mycotoxins in our food could be responsible for millions of cases of mental illness and possibly Autism. There are blood tests to check for food sensitivities and mycotoxins. Government guidelines and scientific studies sometimes offer confusing information. We will discuss some of the controversies in this chapter.

Dietary Guidelines

The USDA provides guidelines based on 2,000 -calories daily intake.

These guidelines are helpful but have been controversial for many years because the people on the Dietary Guidelines Advisory Committee have conflicts of interest and deficient scientific information.

In 1977, the United States, first dietary guidelines recommended fewer animal fats and more grains, replacing most animal fats with industrial processed vegetable oils. Based on a study of 2,467 men who reported identical causes of mortality, these recommendations lacked evidence to support them. Even the new guidelines of 2015 continue to recommend less than 10 percent of calories per day from fats. In the 1980s, the food industry replaced natural fats like butter with harmful trans fats, industrial fats, lard, hydrogenated vegetable oils, and refined sugars to allow the food industry to offer more palatable products. These recommendations were catastrophic. The rate of cardiovascular disease increased, and the mortality rate from heart attacks and strokes skyrocketed. Also, the trends of diabetes, obesity, and cancer increased.

According to the Centers for Disease Control (CDC), 5.19 million people were diagnosed with diabetes in 1978. By 2013, the number had increased to 22.3 million, four times the number 35 years before. In 1970, one in six people was obese. Now, one in two adults is obese, based on a BMI over 30.

Since more people are obese, the rates of cancer have increased despite better treatments. In 1976, the rate of cancer per 100,000 people was 400; by 2016, it was 440.

Death rates from cardiovascular disease have declined due to better treatments and medicine. But they are still very prevalent. The American Heart Association projects that by 2030, over 40 percent of the population will have some form of cardiovascular disease. The tragedy is that cardiovascular disease is preventable and reversible with proper diets.

The problem with the Dietary Guidelines is that they use incorrect hypotheses, and members are under pressure from the food industry to increase profits. Research studies show that diets rich in omega-6 and industrial fats increase the risk of heart disease, as published in the British Medical Journal in 2013.

Refined sugar and the wrong fats caused most of the cardiovascular damage.

Saturated fats raise LDL or bad cholesterol, particularly small, dense LDL. It appears that large fluffy LDL doesn't contribute to heart disease. Studies report that small LDL particles penetrate the arterial wall easily and contribute to forming plaques. Synthetic oils and trans fats penetrate the arterial walls, contributing to plaque formation.

Eating monounsaturated or unsaturated fats like olive and avocado, omega-3 rich in DHA and EPA, and low in omega-6 would be best for a healthier lifestyle. You should avoid industrially refined oils. You must read the labels. Many cakes, cookies, and foods prepared with canola and other refined vegetable oils harm your health. Fast foods, hamburgers, hot dogs, and French fries cooked with industrial oils for hours and days are rich in bad fats, like trans fats and saturated fats. They also contain toxic substances and mycotoxins. I invite you to estimate the number of these harmful foods sold and consumed daily by adding sugary drinks, ice cream, cheeses, dairy, and alcohol. After considering the high levels of fats and carbs in a single meal, you can appreciate the causes and significant problems associated with these diets worldwide. Correcting such a distorted view of feeding ourselves without concern for the potential harm to our organs and life expectancy is mind-boggling. We are facing something similar to what the tobacco industry did with cigarette smoking and the development of lung cancer. All these excesses lead to diseases and morbidity that are preventable. There is no reason for obesity, diabetes, or heart disease to develop if we adopt a wellness lifestyle by eating right and consuming healthy foods and nutrients. Our governments should do more to protect the public by demanding that the food industry eliminate damaging fats, excessive carbohydrates, and chemicals used as fillers, hormones, antibiotics, herbicides, and insecticides in our foods. It is also vital to prevent mycotoxins from mold contaminating foods during harvest and processing by establishing strict controls to lessen the morbidity and mortality associated with silent toxins in our foods.

Keto Diets

For some time, ketogenic diets (KDs), which are low in carbohydrates (less than 5 percent carbs) and rich in fats, have been beneficial to children who have epilepsy or seizure disorders. It also helps children with behavioral disorders, Autism, type 2 diabetes, cancer, and older adults with Alzheimer's and Parkinson's disease (Romanoski 2018). It appears cells learn how to utilize fats faster as a source of energy, decreasing the oxidative process and releasing harmful free radicals, which act as pollutants around the cells.

Keto diets are becoming popular to help people with cancer. Miriam Kalamian, in her book Keto for Cancer, makes a compelling case to assist patients with cancer and benefit from this diet. Through fasting or caloric restriction without malnutrition, it is possible to starve the cancer cells from using carbohydrates to continue their uncontrolled reproduction. This metabolic theory of cancer presents a strong argument that dysfunctional mitochondria are the root cause of initiation and progression of cancer. According to cell biologist Professor Noboru Mizushima, this recycling mechanism, also known as autophagy, is triggered by nutrient starvation. (Mizushima,2007)

Diets to End Coronary Artery Disease and Atherosclerosis

Heart disease is a leading cause of death for men and women in the United States. It claims more deaths than all cancers combined. Obstruction of the coronary arteries causes either sudden death or fatal cardiac arrhythmia. Another problem is the enlargement of the heart caused by high blood pressure. People who die suddenly had no prior warning of heart disease. Most of them die prematurely. Lowering cholesterol and reversing plaque formation and atherosclerosis with diet alone and without medicines should be a goal and will be very beneficial for anyone with a family history of heart disease, evidence of coronary artery disease (CAD) due to genetic factors, bad diets, smoking, and a sedentary lifestyle.

Reversing heart disease, mainly obstruction of the arteries by plaque, has been elusive despite the intake of cholesterol-lowering drugs and medicines to control hypertension.

Research to find the most effective diets to prevent and reverse CAD continues. For many patients, it is frustrating to hear from their cardiologists that there is very little they can do to reverse atherosclerosis and the progression of obstruction of the coronary arteries. It is frightening for many patients to see that, despite losing weight, watching their diets, using cholesterol-lowering drugs, and exercising, the progression of coronary artery disease continues. You can check for increased cardiac calcium scores with a CT angiogram and narrowing of the coronaries to find out. If there is obstruction of a coronary, you should get catheterization for installation of a stent. The technique for this procedure is very advanced; the treatment takes less than an hour without general anesthesia. All these measures, although practical, only provide a few more years of relief from the unavoidable progression of atherosclerosis, heart damage, and ultimate death if you don't follow a strict diet. A plant-based diet is your best option to prevent more plaques or stent obstruction.

A well-known example of the progression of CAD is the case of former Vice President Dick Cheney, who had his first heart attack in his late thirties and multiple attacks after. With the heart so damaged, the only option for Mr. Cheney was a heart transplant. He was lucky to find a new heart and is still alive. He was a very conscientious person and followed his doctor's advice, but he couldn't reverse the progression of atherosclerosis.

The reality is that many patients die of heart disease despite the finest medical care. However, there is hope to reverse atherosclerosis.

In his book, The End of Heart Disease, Joel Fuhrman, MD, has a diet he calls the "Nutritarian diet" to reverse heart disease. Dr. Fuhrman's book is worth reading.

The Standard American Diet (SAD) has proven ineffective in reversing coronary artery disease (CAD).

In 1995, Dr. Caldwell Esselstyn published research demonstrating the reversal of coronary plaque and CAD in seventeen patients with severe CAD. He subsequently expanded his research and demonstrated the reversal of plaque. The study eliminated oils, animal fat, fish, dairy products, and eggs to avoid the formation of trimethylamide oxide (TMAO), an atherogenic compound found in the intestinal flora when consuming animal products. His results were impressive and effective. Many people and researchers find this diet too radical and rigorous. For some people, this diet is challenging to follow. One of the criticisms is the severe restriction of good fats like olive oil, nuts, seeds, and DHA and EPA fat, which may lead to other health problems. To address this, Dr. Furhman recommends the addition of these good fats to his Nutritarian diet, along with low dosages of EPA and DHA fats, to obtain similar results without other health problems due to nutritional deficiencies.

The Pritikin diet

The Pritikin Diet is another plant-based diet that has effectively reversed CAD. Pritikin was only forty-one when he was diagnosed with severe CAD. He developed a diet high in fruits and vegetables and low in oil and animal fats, associated with moderate aerobic exercise. His diet was very effective, and after he died in 1985, an independent autopsy revealed his coronary arteries to be in excellent condition.

The DASH Diet

The DASH diet (Dietary approaches to Stop Hypertension) is designed to prevent hypertension and heart disease. It recommends lower sodium levels (less than 2,400 mg for a standard diet and less than 1,500 mg for a low-sodium diet), whole grains, vegetables, fruits, animal fat, meat, poultry, and dairy products. It is like the Standard American Diet (SAD) but very a significantly low in sodium intake.

The Nutritarian diet

The Nutritarian diet is primarily a plant-based diet rich in micronutrients. This diet includes whole grains, fruits, beans, legumes, nuts, and seeds, allowing for 15 to 25 percent of calories derived from fat. Joel Fuhrman, MD, the creator of this diet, uses an index or ANDI to select foods rich in micronutrients. He ranks foods on a scale of 1 to 1000. Dr. Fuhrman assigns crucíferous leafy greens such as kale and mustard greens with a score of 1000. He also uses a Nutrient IQ score based on portion sizes, which is more practical than using calories. Foods with the highest Nutrient IQ score are vegetables.

The Gundry Diet

Dr. Steven Gundry, in his book The Plant Paradox, raises new questions about the above diets. Dr. Guntry is a heart surgeon who has conducted extensive research on the use of diets and supplements to eliminate heart disease, diabetes, leaky gut syndrome, autoimmune disorders, and many other diseases. The Plant Paradox presents a compelling case about the dangers of certain foods like lectins and WGA (wheat germ agglutinin) lurking on our plates, potentially damaging the coronary arteries and the intestinal wall.

One well-known lectin is gluten, but there are more, causing many problems ignored in many other diets. Take the case of whole grains recommended in different diets. Wheat is the grain that is present in our diets, and it is not our friend, according to Dr. Gundry. He argues that most grains and legumes contain lectins, which trigger an autoimmune response. Lectins also play a role in the obesity crisis. Gundry believes that many people struggle to lose weight if their diets are rich in lectins. Lectins behave like insulin, disrupting the typical passage of sugar inside the cells, causing sugar to turn into fat, resulting in weight gain and insulin resistance.

Gundry suggests that low-carb diets like Atkins or South Beach initially work because they eliminate carbs. But as soon as carbs return, people gain weight. The same is true with the Paleo diet. All these diets have in common is that they initially eliminate lectins to prevent them from acting like insulin and depositing fat in the fat cells. When the lectins return to the diet, they store fat again.

Lectins block sugar from getting inside nerve and muscle cells, interfere with protein digestion, promote inflammation of the mucosal lining of the gut, cross-react with other proteins, cause autoimmune responses, interfere with DNA replication, and contribute to atherosclerosis and plaque formation. One way to avoid WGAs or lectins is to avoid whole-grain bread or products Gundry, 2017, 41–45).

Gundry also reveals that a lectin-binding sugar, called Neu5Ac, sits in the lining of the arteries and cells in the gut wall. We share this molecule with elephants, who are also affected by the same problem. Other species, including chimps and gorillas, can't make this molecule and don't get atherosclerosis like humans and elephants. They have a slightly different molecule called Neu5Gc, which doesn't bind with grain lectins.

When humans consume red meat, which contains Neu5Gc, our immune system recognizes that this molecule is different. Our white cells react by producing antibodies that attach to the lining of our blood vessels, which have Neu5Ac. This mistaken attack by our immune system damages the lining of our coronaries, leading to the development of atherosclerosis (Gundry 2017, 154–59).

Gundry recommends removing lectins by:

1) Soaking beans and legumes, including grains, before eating them.
2) Pressure cooking. Using a pressure cooker is the best way to eliminate lectins.
3) Peel and deseed. Removing the seeds of plant foods such as cucumbers, eggplant, squash, and tomatoes.

4) Fermenting. When you ferment a fruit or a vegetable, you allow good bacteria to break down and convert lectins into healthier foods. He also recommends removing the brown rice hull and cauliflower rice as an alternative to rice.

Lectins are proteins found mainly in legumes and grains, but with good preparation, a lectin-free diet is possible.

In his book *"How Not to Age,"* Dr. Michael Greger recommends legumes like beans, lentils, and whole grains. His book provides extensive studies backing the benefits of legumes. The *Blue Zones* book also includes information on different centenarian populations who consume legumes regularly.

Though quality research is limited, its suggests that lectins may cause poor digestion, inflammation, and various diseases in some people sensitive to legumes and gluten.

Soaking and cooking legumes seem to diminish these problems since they are an excellent source of nutrients and antioxidants.

Much scientific research now points to a plant-based diet with low or non-animal fats to extend life and be more favorable to healthy longevity. We have to become selective with all the fats we consume. A plant-based diet must add fish and more omega-3 than omega-6 with proportional higher levels of DHA and EPA.

Paleo Diets

A paleo diet refers to foods that humans might have eaten during the Paleolithic Era, which lasted from around 2.5 million to 10,000 years ago.

A modern paleo diet includes fruits, vegetables, lean meats, fish, eggs, nuts and seeds. These are foods that, in the past, people could get by hunting and gathering. It excludes foods that became more common when small-scale farming began about 10,000 years ago, such as grains, legumes, and dairy products.

Paleo diets are essentially low-carb and high-protein diets. The Paleo diet allows meats and eggs, rich in saturated fats. High protein diets also contain too much methionine and BCAA (Branch Chain Amino Acids), which are unhealthy. I don't recommend these diets because no scientific research supports them. The fact our ancestors ate these foods doesn't mean they were very knowledgeable in nutrition and their role in improving our health. The only point that is widely acceptable is that humans millions of years ago were primarily vegetarians or vegans. Animals, apes, and herbivores develop pretty nicely with a plant-based diet. We see the same in wild animals like buffaloes, elephants, cattle, and horses without significant deficiencies. Today, we understand the role of proteins, fats, sugars, amino acids, and vitamins and the contributions of our microbiome to improving our health and longevity. Living longer than our ancestors 100 years ago is a testament to our growing knowledge about nutrients. But we need to learn more. We are just scratching the surface. With the help of technology, AI, and quantum computing, we will understand the chemical processes happening at the cellular level in real time in the following decades. If humans begin to populate the planets, a deep knowledge of our chemical structure and functions is necessary to survive where no plants are available. Plants that can survive and adapt to an adverse environment will provide the nutrients to all future planetary explorers.

How Do Toxins in Our Diets Affect Health and Longevity?

By testing for IgG antibodies in the blood, we can detect which food we are sensitive to. Specialized labs can detect many food sensitivities with one sample. Some labs offer testing for hundreds of foods with one sample. Also, testing for molds or mycotoxins is possible with the same sample. Mycotoxins act as anti-nutrients. Mold is challenging to detect because, during the process, it mixes with regular food. The toxins, however, stay in food during the processing and preparation without our knowledge. Mold and mycotoxins grow in exposed grains like coffee beans, legumes, corn, wheat, peanuts, nuts, fruits, wine, chocolate, milk, cheeses, corn-fed animals, and fish. Peeled onions and garlic in our refrigerators also get contaminated with mold.

Mycotoxins continue in the food until food is ready to eat. If you feel sick after eating some foods, you will most likely continue with mycotoxins or additives during processing. Prolonged exposure to mycotoxins can trigger chronic inflammation, raising cytokines until we develop organ damage. Examples are autoimmune disorders like lupus and rheumatoid arthritis, out of dozens of inflammatory diseases. Most recent mental illness is also within this group. Medications also get contaminated with mycotoxins. In 2012, cortisone injectable became infected with a fungus. More than 200 people got sick, and 16 died just after the injection. The drug became contaminated in the lab of a compound pharmacy. Mold can also grow in homes where humidity is high, leading to people breathing in the spores and swallowing the mucous, resulting in illnesses.

Unfortunately, medical education doesn't prepare doctors to diagnose and treat these problems. Nutrition and food contamination are not part of the medical curriculum. In my practice, I often encountered patients on benzodiazepines, opioids, and tranquilizers for the symptoms listed above. In reality, further testing to identify food sensitivity or mycotoxins provided the answer. Patients got better without needing medications by eliminating the offensive agents or toxins.

As children grow up or if we have an active life and exercise, we may need additional nutrients like amino acids, vitamins, minerals, or supplements. Deficiencies of nutrients are particularly evident as we age. Our cells, over time, decline, and many die. The result is the loss of hormones or nutrients to maintain all our cells healthy and well-nourished. Medicines may interfere with the absorption of nutrients or cause deficiencies at the cellular level. Adding supplements to compensate for these deficiencies may be necessary. In the next chapter, we will explore the role of nutrition and supplements in promoting optimal health.

CHAPTER 4

Vitamins, Probiotics, Prebiotics, Minerals, and Supplements

Many diets don't have all the minerals and nutrients necessary for good nutrition. Many diets lack probiotics, prebiotics, minerals, and other essential chemicals for a better and more balanced function of the cells. Without the proper ingredients, the cells that work as tiny factories 24 hours a day- cannot produce the neurotransmitter, hormone, or protein for an essential function by the recipient cells in the production chain. With deficiencies, the entire body and all its systems are in trouble. Think about a factory that makes cookies. They need flour, sugar, eggs, baking soda, salt, fats, milk and other ingredients. If sugar or any other ingredient is unavailable, the cookies produced will be of poor quality and rejected by the buyer. A similar situation occurs at the cellular level.

Recent research suggests that imbalances in gut microbiota may be responsible for these deficiencies. There is a strong connection between the gut microbiota and the brain. Deficiency of some bacteria in the intestine may lead to many neurological disorders. Adding these bacteria improves neurological function. Studies in patients with Parkinson's disease and Autism suggest a strong correlation exists when some bacteria like Lactobacillus plantarum are present in a diet, cognitive and neurological function improves. We will consider some of these cases ahead of time in a subtitle about probiotics.

Some vitamins, minerals, and nutrients are essential for cellular function since the body doesn't produce them. One of the most critical properties of modern dietary supplements is their ease of absorption or bioavailability. Without good absorption, the efficacy is limited. Many active ingredients/nutrients are lipophilic (fat-soluble) or insoluble in water, consequently offering poor bioavailability.

When selecting vitamins, you should pay attention to their absorption to maximize their benefits. Our bodies need daily fatty acids, vitamins, and minerals for optimal function and balance.

Essential fatty acids like omega-3 are necessary to make cell membranes and repair tissues daily. Vitamin C is another example. The same is true for many minerals, like iodine and iron. Iodine deficiencies cause goiter, and iron deficiencies cause anemia. Folic acid is a vitamin that may be deficient in many women. A deficiency of folic acid in a pregnant woman may cause brain and neurological damage to the unborn child. Some diets lack vitamins or minerals and require additional supplements. Parents should know that children reared on soda pop, fries, and pizza do not get enough nutrients and vitamins. The same is true for many women during pregnancy. In addition, as a person ages, most cells do not get enough nutrients due to medications, absorption problems, or bad diets. To be balanced and play it safe, taking a multivitamin with minerals every day is better. In excess, specific vitamins and minerals are detrimental.

Some examples are 1) Iron, 2) Folic acid, 3) vitamins A and E. 4) copper, calcium, and iodine. You most likely don't need more vitamins with a balanced diet. Still, you will benefit from extra vitamins and minerals if you have absorption problems, anemia, or thyroid deficiencies.

Many over-the-counter (OTC) medications can also deplete vital nutrients. For example, aspirin depletes iron, folic acid, vitamin C, and potassium, while NSAIDs deplete DHEA, folic acid, melatonin, and zinc. Common prescription drugs, like statin drugs to lower cholesterol, deplete CoQ10 and vitamins D and E. Corticosteroids, usually taken for inflammation, deplete calcium, magnesium, zinc, selenium, potassium, DHEA, vitamins C and

D, and folic acid. Contraceptives deplete B complex vitamins, magnesium, zinc, tyrosine, and vitamin C. In the following paragraphs, I will go into more detail about the vitamins' properties and the interaction and side effects of some vitamins and minerals.

Are Autism and other neurological disorders like Parkinson's Disease, Chronic Anxiety, and Depression Linked to Gut Problems?

Recent research suggests a strong correlation between a deficiency of neurotransmitters and a deficiency of some bacteria in our microbiota.

Autism Spectrum Disorder is a neurodevelopmental disorder. Recent data suggest that probiotics can reduce some symptoms of this disorder, and Lactobacillus plantarum PS128 is especially useful. Researchers recruited a sample of 131 autistic children and adolescents. They evaluated their changes after the use of probiotics using CGI. They found some significant improvements with few side effects; these positive effects were more evident in younger children. Patients taking Lactobacillus plantarum PS128 had more significant improvements and fewer side effects than those taking other probiotics. Their data is consistent with existing literature showing a specific effect of Lactobacillus plantarum PS128 in Autism Spectrum Disorder. Other studies in Parkinson's patients have demonstrated improved cognitive and motor function. It appears that the levels of dopamine and serotonin increase for improved neurotransmission—the probiotic acts as the factory, making the neurotransmitter that is deficient at the cellular level.

Another group of patients who may benefit from this probiotic are persons suffering from depression and persistent anxiety. Studies in this group of patients show improvement due to the increased dopamine and serotonin at the intestinal level by the Lactobacillus Plantarum PS128. One observation from this study is why the levels of dopamine and serotonin decrease, leading to these neurological disorders. Antibiotics may be responsible for losing Lactobacillus Plantarum and other valuable probiotics. Replacing the probiotic helps to restore a balanced microbiota and, in particular, these helpful probiotics. More studies are necessary to test this theory. In the meantime, it is useful for any doctor or patient to realize that if a person develops anxiety or depression after using antibiotics, the cause is very likely the killing of this necessary probiotic. Children who have Autism or behavioral disorders could benefit from treatment with this probiotic to restore a healthy microbiota, particularly after treatment with antibiotics. Parents must become aware that frequent use of antibiotics is unhealthy since they kill most of the good bacteria in the gut and promote the growth of harmful bacteria with more severe consequences. A parent with an autistic child must request a test to identify all bacteria in the feces of the child. Today, many laboratories provide a complete list of all the good and bad probiotics in the microbiota, as well as mycotoxins, worms, fungi, and other obnoxious organisms.

Vitamins, Minerals, and Supplements

Can inflammation affect the absorption of vitamins and minerals?

Inflammation is responsible for absorption problems and malnutrition. Many people are sensitive to many foods. Others have serious allergies, causing severe inflammatory responses along the intestinal wall. Some foods enhance or decrease the absorption of vitamins. Food allergies and sensitivities like gluten and WGA, present in wheat and other foods, may cause gut inflammation, affecting the absorption of minerals, vitamins, and other nutrients. Some foods trigger the elevation of zonulin, which increases intestinal permeability, leading to autoimmune disorders. Some vitamins and minerals are essential for the gut bacteria or microbiota to process foods properly.

Too much calcium can impair iron absorption, while vitamin C, for example, increases it. Calcium and magnesium compete for absorption. It is better to take them separately. I recommend taking 400 mg of magnesium in the evening or before sleep. It helps the body to relax. B complex vitamins are water-soluble, so taking them in the morning is better.

The fat-soluble vitamins like A, D, E, and K) are best taken with a fatty meal. Most supplements typically work better before breakfast or two hours apart from meals.

In Appendix A, I have listed my morning essentials, which are a smoothie containing vitamin C and omega-3. You can add other nutrients while you enjoy this delicious smoothie. I usually take this smoothie with my B complex, CoQ10, alpha lipoic acid, glutamine, NMN, NAC, Vitamin D, and zinc. If you establish a routine, you will not miss your daily supplements.

Years ago, my wife developed swelling of the joints of both hands. After trying different treatments unsuccessfully, she found a combination of supplements that relieved the swelling. My wife now takes Turmeric (curcumin caps), glucosamine, SAM-e, Boswellia, and omega-3 daily to decrease inflammation of her hands' joints. She found this combination the best to control persistent pain and swelling of her hands. This combination effectively reduced inflammation and pain, a solution I now recommend to my patients.

After this experience, I began recommending a combination of these nutrients and supplements to my patients, with good results.

Many people are unaware of the analgesic and anti-inflammatory benefits of supplements. The FDA prohibits advertising these benefits because they don't meet the rigorous testing of many pharmaceuticals. The fact is that many supplements have been around for thousands of years, and many drugs come from synthetic chemicals that provide similar beneficial effects to the natural chemicals found in many herbs and supplements.

In my experience, many supplements alone or combined help relieve inflammation and pain. For example, omega-3, SAM-e, and Turmeric are safe and reasonable pain relievers.

If you feel deficient in any nutrient or vitamin, you should ask your doctor to do a test. Many national laboratories offer tests for minerals and vitamins. Unfortunately, many doctors are unaware —or not interested—about how nutrition works to heal and the harmful effects medications cause, preventing the absorption of nutrients and minerals. Their focus is on the prescribed medicine, not the disruption of the cellular level's balance of nutrients, vitamins, and minerals.

If you are tired or without energy, many doctors prefer to give you an antidepressant when the problem could be low magnesium or a vitamin D deficiency. Fortunately, there are labs today where you can get your lab work without a doctor's prescription.

You can find in Appendix B a list of laboratories that offer testing for all these minerals and vitamins and genetic testing when contacted directly. If any test is abnormal and your doctor shows no interest, you should look for a doctor interested in nutritional deficiencies or hormone problems. Searching the internet, you will find doctors in your area whom you can contact to address specific issues. Doctors specializing in comprehensive integrative, alternative medicine, functional medicine, or lifestyle medicine offer counseling in nutrition and alternative forms of treatment.

When you shop at the supermarket, always look for fresh vegetables and fruits. Fruits and vegetables contain phytochemicals, polyphenols, antioxidants, flavonoids, and nutrients that protect against cancer, heart disease, and many chronic diseases. Among the most potent phytochemicals are pigments such as chlorophyll, carotene, and flavonoids found in a rainbow assortment of fruits and vegetables. Other phytochemicals include dietary fiber, enzymes, oils, and vitamin-like compounds. Fiber is essential to keep your gut bacteria working for your benefit and control carbohydrate absorption. Fiber acts as a prebiotic, which is vital for digestion.

Phytochemicals work harmoniously with essential nutrients such as vitamin C, E, B complex vitamins, zinc, selenium, omega-3 fatty acids, CoQ10, and many other compounds to exert considerably greater protection. They also work as antioxidants to protect against oxidative damage from free radicals responsible for DNA damage. Ironically, the oxygen molecule is the primary source of free radicals and oxidative damage in the body. The molecule that gives us life is also the molecule that can cause the most harm. Oxidative and free radical damage is the primary cause of aging. Free radicals contribute to the development of cancers, heart disease, cataracts, Alzheimer's disease, arthritis, chronic inflammation, and many other degenerative diseases.

The environment also contributes significantly to the free radical load that damages the cells. Cigarette smoking substantially increases the free radical load and causes significant damage. The harmful effects of smoking are related to the high levels of free radicals inhaled, depleting essential antioxidants such as vitamin C and beta-carotene. Other external sources of free radicals include ionizing radiation, drugs, air pollutants, pesticides, anesthetics, aromatic hydrocarbons, fried foods, solvents, alcohol, formaldehyde, and many other products used in the home and food processing.

In conclusion, free radicals constantly bombard all humans and they should find protection with a diet rich in vegetables and fruits. The antioxidants in plant-based foods protect us against free radicals and oxidative damage. Taking supplements can help to fight the damage done by these free radicals.

Vitamin A

Vitamin A is essential for vision and for activating the immune system. Activated vitamin A turns into retinol, which is used in creams to reduce wrinkles. Using these creams during the day is not recommended since retinol may accelerate the development of skin cancer when exposed to the sun. Some prescription drugs for acne (Accutane) and psoriasis (Soriatane) contain synthetic forms of retinol and are very dangerous during pregnancy because they can cause congenital disabilities. Retinol integrates with iron and hemoglobin in the bones to carry oxygen to the cells.

Conditions that interfere with normal digestion can lead to vitamin A malabsorption, such as celiac disease, Crohn's disease, cirrhosis, alcoholism, and cystic fibrosis. Also at risk are adults and children with nutritional deficits in their diets due to poverty or self-restriction. Mild vitamin A deficiency may result in fatigue, infection susceptibility, and infertility. Severe deficiencies may present as:

1. Xerophthalmia (severe dryness of the eye which can lead to blindness if not treated.
2. Nyctalopia or night blindness
3. Irregular patches on the whites of the eyes
4. Dry skin or hair

Too much vitamin A may be harmful for people who smoke since it predisposes some people to lung cancer. Studies show a 28 percent increase in the rate of lung cancer in people taking vitamin A. The death rate from heart disease increases to 17 percent with beta-carotenes.

Another cancer associated with the intake of beta-carotene is prostate cancer.

In contrast to preformed vitamin A, beta-carotene is not toxic even at high intake levels. The body can form vitamin A from beta-carotene as needed, and there is no need to monitor intake levels as with preformed vitamin A. Therefore, it is preferable to choose a multivitamin supplement that has all or the vast majority of its vitamin A in the form of beta-carotene; many multivitamin manufacturers have already reduced the amount of preformed vitamin A in their products. However, most people have no solid reason to take individual high-dose beta-carotene supplements.

Smokers, in particular, should avoid vitamin A supplements since some randomized trials in smokers have linked high-dose supplements with increased lung cancer risk. Several studies have found an association between increased mortality rate and beta-carotene supplementation.

I do not recommend vitamin A if you eat a healthy diet that contains carotenes, which are present in colorful fruits and vegetables. A multivitamin containing no more than 3,000 IU of vitamin A is safe for men and 2000 IU for women. Pregnant women should not take more than 3,000 IU a day.

B complex vitamins

Table 3. B complex vitamins

Vitamin B1	Thiamine	Involved in metabolism of sugars and amino acids	Present in whole grains, brown rice, whole green diets, poultry, fish, eggs, pork, shellfish, wheat pasta, yeast, peas
Vitamin B2	Riboflavin	Cofactor of flavoprotein reactions and vitamins	Present in yeast extract, whole grains, liver, cheese
Vitamin B3	Niacin	Precursor of NAD and NADP for many metabolic processes	Present in lean meat, whole grains, brewer's yeast, cheese, fish, eggs, whole wheat bread
Vitamin B5	Pantothenic acid	Precursor of coenzyme A and other molecules	Present in brewer's yeast, royal jelly, liver, nuts, whole grains, eggs
Vitamin B6	Pyridoxine	Coenzyme of many metabolic reactions	Present in wheat germ, bananas, chicken, fish, potatoes, Brussels sprouts, whole wheat bread, green vegetables
Vitamin B7	Biotin	Involved in fatty acids synthesis and gluconeogenesis	Present in peanuts, almonds, eggs yolks, walnuts, chicken, sesame seeds
Vitamin B9	Folic acid	Precursor to make and repair DNA; helps cell division and growth during pregnancy	Present in green diets, poultry, fish, eggs, pork, shellfish
Vitamin B12	Cobalamins, cyanocobalamins, and methylcobalamins	Involved in metabolism of all cells, affecting DNA synthesis and regulation; also involved in fatty acid and amino acid metabolism	Present in liver, beef, pork, fish, eggs, yeast, milk; not found in plants, and vegans may develop a deficiency

These are among my favorite vitamins. Several vitamins are in this group. They work synergistically to protect the cardiovascular, skeletal, and nervous systems. I have listed them in Table 3 with information about their actions. B6, B12, and B9 are involved in formation of red cells. They also protect the heart against the actions of homocysteine and play a significant role in DNA methylation. Most vegetables and fruits have these vitamins, except for B12. Vegetarians who do not consume eggs, fish, or animal food are deficient in this crucial vitamin. Biotin (vitamin 7) is a popular vitamin marketed to improve hair health or prevent alopecia. To date, there is a lack of published studies to suggest that biotin supplements benefit the growth of normal, healthy hair and nails.

Despite the inconclusive evidence, biotin supplements remain popular. Between 1999 and 2016, the proportion of supplement users increased nearly thirtyfold. In November 2017, the US Food and Drug Administration (FDA) issued a warning based on reports of biotin supplements interfering with laboratory blood tests, causing incorrect results. High doses have produced either falsely elevated or decreased blood levels, depending on the test. Such dosages of biotin have affected lab results of certain hormones, such as thyroid-stimulating hormone and Vitamin D, as well as a biomarker for heart attacks called troponin. Case reports of this occurrence showed people taking biotin amounts much higher than the AIAI level (30 micrograms daily or 0.03 mg) but in doses commonly found in supplements (10-300 mg). Biotin is present in multivitamins and hair/nail/skin supplements.

Folate is the natural form of vitamin B9, water-soluble, and naturally found in many foods. It is also added to foods and sold as a supplement in folic acid; this form is better when coming from food sources—85% vs. 50%, respectively. Folate helps to form DNA and RNA and is involved in protein metabolism. It plays a crucial role in breaking down homocysteine, an amino acid that can exert harm if present in high amounts. Folate is also needed to produce healthy red blood cells and is critical during periods of rapid growth, such as during pregnancy and fetal development.

The Recommended Dietary Allowance (RDA) for folate is measured in micrograms (mcg) of dietary folate equivalents (DFE).

Men and women ages 19 years and older should aim for 400 mcg DFE. Pregnant and lactating women require 600 mcg DFE and 500 mcg DFE, respectively. People who regularly drink alcohol should aim for at least 600 mcg DFE of folate daily since alcohol can impair its absorption.

Folic acid also helps to decrease the levels of homocysteine, an amino acid responsible for increasing the risk factors for heart disease. A deficiency of folic acid also leads to anemia, loss of cognitive function in children and older adults, hearing loss, skin patches like vitiligo, and slow growth in children.

Deficiencies also develop with malabsorption syndromes like Crohn's disease, celiac syndrome, alcoholism, and kidney dialysis. It affects the medication intake of Dilantin, methotrexate, and sulfa.

Good sources of folate include:

- Dark green leafy vegetables (turnip greens, spinach, romaine lettuce, asparagus, Brussel sprouts, broccoli)
- Beans
- Peanuts
- Sunflower seeds
- Fruits, fruit juices
- Whole grains
- Liver
- Fish
- Eggs
- Fortified foods and supplements

Vitamin B12, or cobalamin, is naturally found in animal foods and is present in many fortified foods or supplements. It is needed to form red blood cells and DNA as long as the key function and development of brain and nerve cells.

Vitamin B12 binds to the protein in the foods we eat. Hydrochloric acid and enzymes unbind vitamin B12 into its free form in the stomach. From there, vitamin B12 combines with an intrinsic factor protein to be absorbed further in the small intestine.

Supplements and fortified foods contain B12 in its free form so that they may be more easily absorbed. There is a variety of vitamin B12 supplements available. Although there are claims that certain forms of sublingual tablets or liquids placed under the tongue have better absorption than traditional tablets, studies have not shown a critical difference. Vitamin B12 tablets are available in high dosages, far above the recommended dietary allowance. Still, these high amounts are unnecessary because an adequate intrinsic factor is also needed. In cases of severe vitamin B12 deficiency due to inadequate levels of intrinsic factor (pernicious anemia), doctors may prescribe B12 injections in the muscle.

The Recommended Dietary Allowance for men and women ages 14 years and older is 2.4 micrograms (mcg) daily. The amount increases to 2.6 and 2.8 mcg daily for pregnancy and lactation, respectively.

Food Sources

- Fish and shellfish
- Liver
- Red meat
- Eggs
- Poultry
- Dairy products
- Fortified nutritional yeast
- Fortified breakfast cereals
- Enriched soy or rice milk

Vitamin B12 Deficiency

Measuring vitamin B12 in the blood is not the best way to determine whether someone is deficient, as some people with a deficiency can show normal B12 blood levels. Blood levels of *methylmalonic acid,* a protein breakdown product, and homocysteine are better markers that capture actual vitamin B12 activity. These values increase with a vitamin B12 deficiency. Up to 15% of the general population is estimated to have a vitamin B12 deficiency.

Factors that may cause vitamin B12 deficiency:

- **Avoiding animal products.** People who do not eat meat, fish, poultry, or dairy are at risk of becoming deficient in vitamin B12 since it is only found naturally in animal products. Studies have shown that vegetarians have low vitamin B blood levels. For this reason, those who follow a vegetarian or vegan diet should include B12-fortified foods or a B12 supplement. It is vital for pregnant women, as the fetus requires adequate vitamin B12 for neurologic development, and a deficiency can lead to permanent neurological damage in the fetus.
- **Lack of intrinsic factor.** Pernicious anemia is an autoimmune disease that attacks and potentially destroys gut cells so that levels of **intrinsic factors** are not present, which is crucial for vitamin B12 to be absorbed. If vitamin B12 deficiency ensues, other types of anemia and neurological damage may result. Even a high-dose B12 supplement will not solve the problem, as the **intrinsic factor** is not absorbed.
- **Inadequate stomach acid.** A more common cause of B12 deficiency, especially in older people, is a lack of stomach acid because stomach acid is needed to liberate vitamin B12 from food. Approximately 10-30% of adults over 50 have difficulty absorbing vitamin B12 from food. People who regularly take medications that suppress stomach acid for conditions like gastroesophageal reflux disease (GERD) or peptic ulcer disease—such as proton-pump inhibitors, H2 blockers, or other antacids—may have difficulty absorbing vitamin B12 from food. These drugs can slow the release or decrease the production of stomach acid. In theory, this can prevent the vitamin from being released into its free usable form in the stomach; however, research has not shown an increased prevalence of a deficiency in people using these medications. Anyone using these medications for an extended time and who is at risk for a vitamin B12 deficiency for other reasons should be monitored closely by their physician. They may also use fortified foods or

supplements with vitamin B12, as these forms are typically absorbed well and do not require stomach acid.
- **Intestinal surgeries or digestive disorders that cause malabsorption.** Surgeries that remove the stomach, where intrinsic factor is produced, or the ileum (the last portion of the small intestine), where vitamin B12 is absorbed, develop the risk of a deficiency. Certain diseases, including Crohn's and celiac disease that negatively impact the digestive tract, also increase the risk of deficiency.
- Long-term use of metformin, a drug commonly prescribed for type 2 diabetes, is strongly associated with vitamin B12 deficiency and lower folic acid levels as it can block absorption. This may lead to increased homocysteine levels and a risk for cardiovascular disease. Proton pump inhibitors and histamine blockers prescribed to reduce stomach acid are also associated with lower vitamin B12 levels and the risk of stomach cancer.

Signs of deficiency may include:

- Megaloblastic anemia—a condition of more significant than average-sized red blood cells and a smaller than usual amount; this occurs because there is not enough vitamin B12 in the diet or poor absorption
- Pernicious anemia—a type of megaloblastic anemia caused by a lack of intrinsic factors so that vitamin B12 is not absorbed
- Fatigue, weakness
- Nerve damage causing numbness and tingling in the hands and legs
- Memory loss, confusion
- Dementia
- Depression
- Seizures

B vitamin complex supplements are frequently marketed to boost energy levels and mood. People with a B vitamin deficiency may feel a rise in energy levels after using the supplement because the vitamin is directly involved in making healthy blood cells and can correct anemia if present. However, there is no evidence of benefit if people without a deficiency take extra B vitamins.

- People who eat a vegan diet believe Brewer's or nutritional yeast contains B12. However, yeast does not naturally contain this vitamin and will only be present if fortified with it. Be aware that certain brands, but not all, contain B12.
- Nori (purple laver), the dried edible seaweed used to make sushi rolls, is sometimes promoted as a plant source of vitamin B12. It does contain small amounts of active vitamin B12, but the amount varies among types of seaweed, with some containing none. Therefore, it is not considered a reliable food source.

Vitamin C

Vitamin C (ascorbic acid) is an essential nutrient needed for forming blood vessels, cartilage, muscle, and collagen in soft tissues to prevent wrinkles. It is also essential in the nervous, immune, blood, and bones. Vitamin C is also vital to your body's healing process.

Vitamin C is an antioxidant that helps protect your cells against the effects of free radicals — molecules produced when your body breaks down food or from tobacco smoke and radiation from the sun, X-rays, or other sources. Free radicals might play a role in heart disease, cancer, and other diseases. Vitamin C also helps your body absorb and store iron.

Because your body doesn't produce vitamin C, you must get it from your diet. Vitamin C is present in citrus fruits, berries, potatoes, tomatoes, peppers, cabbage, Brussels sprouts, broccoli, and spinach. Vitamin C is also available as an oral supplement, typically in capsules and chewable tablets.

Most people get enough vitamin C from a healthy diet. Vitamin C deficiency is more likely in people who:

- Smoke or are exposed to secondhand smoking
- Have certain gastrointestinal conditions or certain types of cancer
- Have a limited diet that doesn't regularly include fruits and vegetables

Severe vitamin C deficiency can lead to scurvy, which causes anemia, bleeding gums, and bruising.

If you take vitamin C for its antioxidant properties, remember that the supplement might not offer the same benefits as naturally occurring antioxidants in food.

The recommended daily amount of vitamin C is 90 milligrams for adult men and 75 milligrams for adult women.

If you take vitamin C for its antioxidant properties, remember that the supplement might not offer the same benefits as naturally occurring antioxidants in food.

- Vitamin C improves the absorption of nonheme iron, which is present in plant foods such as leafy greens. Drinking a small glass of 100% fruit juice or including a vitamin-C-rich food with meals can help boost iron absorption.
- Vitamin C can be destroyed by heat and light. High-heat cooking temperatures or prolonged cook times can break down the vitamin. Because it is water-soluble, the vitamin can also seep into cooking liquid. You should try quick heating methods or use as little water as possible when cooking, such as stir-frying or blanching, as these can preserve the vitamin. Foods at peak ripeness eaten raw contain the most vitamin C.
- Vitamin C serums and skin creams are popular because normal skin typically contains high concentrations of vitamin C, which stimulates collagen production and protects against UV sunlight damage. However, research suggests that topical vitamin C may have limited benefits, as very little can penetrate the skin's surface and will not produce additional benefits if a person obtains adequate vitamin C through food or supplements.

Vitamin D

Vitamin D deficiency is a real problem in regions of the country where there is little exposure to the sun. In tropical countries, a few minutes of sunlight increases vitamin D levels significantly. In contrast, in northern countries or states away from the equator, particularly during the winter, the lack of the sun reduces vitamin D levels, predisposing people to many illnesses. A dosage of 2,000 IU of vitamin D is appropriate for most people in these areas. In areas with more sun, I recommend 1,000 IU once or twice a day depending on the person's level of Vitamin D. If the blood level of vitamin D3 is below 30 mg/ml, a vitamin D3 supplementation is recommended. Good food sources of vitamin D include milk, orange juice, fish, salmon, sardines, fish liver oils, eggs, beef, and butter. Some studies have found an association between multiple sclerosis (MSMS) and neuromuscular diseases with Vitamin D deficiencies.

Many other diseases and health problems are associated with vitamin D deficiency. These include osteomalacia and bone deformities in children, atopic dermatitis, inflammatory bowel disease, asthmatic attacks, cardiovascular problems, sudden cardiac death, cancer of the pancreas, fertility problems, and low testosterone in men with erectile dysfunction. Vitamin D affects about 3,000 genes and is essential in preventing many health problems and maintaining optimal health. Low levels of 25-hydroxy vitamin D are associated with erectile dysfunction, hypogonadism, and fertility problems in hypogonadal men.

Vitamin D also raises estradiol levels in men and women and helps prevent osteoporosis by increasing bone mass. Some ongoing studies are also exploring the use of vitamin D in preventing pancreatic cancer.

The micronutrient works through the microbiome by increasing the levels of the bacterium Bacteroides fragilis, which improves the cancer immune response.

Sunscreen decreases the production of vitamin D; for example, a cream with an SPF of 8 can lower the production of vitamin D by 95 percent. It is important to achieve a balance since sunscreen protects against damaging UVUV rays that cause skin cancer and wrinkles. I recommend having your vitamin D levels checked by a doctor to see if you are deficient in this essential vitamin. If so, you may then consider vitamin D supplementation.

Vitamin E

Vitamin E is an essential nutrient that helps maintain the health and function of the reproductive, vascular, and neuromuscular systems. This vitamin is an excellent antioxidant and reduces the damage caused by free radicals. Vitamin E also helps prevent damage to the DNA due to oxidative stress. Since inflammation is associated with cardiovascular problems, diabetes, arthritis, and cancer, supplementation with vitamin E, particularly in the forms of alpha-tocopherol and gamma-tocopherol, significantly helps reduce inflammation.

Many scientific studies confirm these findings. For example, the American Cancer Society, in a survey of more than a million adults, found that those who regularly take 200 IU of vitamin E each day have a lower risk of developing bladder cancer. Another study, the SELECT (Selenium and Vitamin E Cancer Prevention Trial), looked at 35,000 men taking 400 IU of vitamin E and found that there was an increase in prostate cancer. For this reason, it is generally recommended not to take more than 200 IU of vitamin E (NIH Office of Dietary Supplements 2018).

In a study conducted on veterans at numerous VAVA centers, vitamin E decreases the development of dementia and Alzheimer's disease and the decline in cognitive function as we age. Women going through menopause and experiencing hot flashes who take between 600 and 800 IU of vitamin E have significant benefits. Several studies cite the benefits of vitamin E to improve fertility in males. Vitamin E is vital to maintain healthy skin, hair, and nails. Always check Vitamin E, an ingredient in many creams and lotions (LowDog 2016, 134–40).

The best dietary sources of vitamin E are sunflower seeds, almonds, spinach, fish, eggs, avocados, green leafy vegetables, vegetable oils, olive oil, and wheat germ.

Prolonged vitamin E deficiency may increase the risk of peripheral neuropathy, infection, anemia, and problems for the mother and baby during pregnancy. A multivitamin that provides at least 30 IUIU of vitamin E is adequate. Generally, dosages greater than 100 IU are unnecessary with a proper diet. Vitamin E depends on selenium, copper, zinc, and manganese as supplementation.

Some individuals, especially those with Crohn's disease, cystic fibrosis, or a genetic disorder known as abetalipoproteinemia (which affects the absorption of dietary fats, cholesterol, and fat-soluble vitamins), may require vitamin E supplementation

Vitamin K

Vitamin K deficiency causes symptoms such as bleeding of the gums, nosebleeds, easy bruising, and heavy menstrual periods. Individuals at higher risk of vitamin K deficiency include alcoholics and people with digestive disorders that impair fat absorption, such as Crohn's disease, cystic fibrosis, and other intestinal conditions. A diet rich in green leafy vegetables is a good source of vitamin K. A cup of kale provides 1,000 mcg of K1. In contrast, spinach, lettuce, turnip greens, avocado, cheeses, and kiwi fruits help to raise vitamin K levels to carboxylate osteocalcin, improving bone quality.

If supplementation is needed, a dose from 150 to 300 mcg daily is adequate. The dosage recommended of K2 as MK-4 is 500 mcg per day. The subtypes MK-4 and MK-7 are the best for human health. Supplementation can be effective in reducing plaques in coronary arteries. Taking MK-7 for six months lowers plaque and calcium scores. K2 supplementation is crucial if you have cardiovascular disease, diabetes, or are at risk of osteoporosis or prostate cancer.

Vitamin K2 also helps transport calcium to the proper areas of the body. A deficiency of vitamin K2 is the possible cause of calcification of the arteries. The Rotterdam study of 7,983 men and women found that K2, but not K1, has a strong protective effect. There was a reduction in arterial calcification and death when the subjects ate foods rich in K2. Two famous longitudinal studies, the Nurses' Health Study and the Framingham Heart

Study, found that people with low dietary vitamin K intake have a greater risk of hip fractures. The lack of carboxylation of this bone-building protein, osteocalcin, is at the root of the fractures. K1 and K2 increase carboxylation of osteocalcin, making bones stronger. Research shows that taking vitamins K and D, calcium, and magnesium keeps bones more robust and prevents osteoporosis and osteoporosis. However, individuals taking warfarin (Coumadin) to prevent blood clots should avoid Vitamin K supplementation.

Minerals

Minerals are necessary for many chemical reactions to allow many cells to perform their metabolic functions. Along with amino acids, vitamins, and other chemicals, cells need minerals to complete their jobs. Material management is a factory process that is not different from that of a manufacturer that needs different elements like gold, silver, or copper to finish a product. A lack of one or two elements may produce an inferior product, resulting in a defective outcome. Fortunately, most vegetables and fruits contain enough minerals to maintain a balanced diet. Below is a list of some of the most critical minerals for better health.

Regarding minerals, I do not recommend extra iron intake unless you are anemic, pregnant, or have low thyroid, and testing indicates you are deficient in iron. Too much iron may be toxic, and the same is true with some other minerals.

Copper is another mineral that requires careful monitoring. Excess copper may reduce immune function and increase mental decline. It helps transport iron to the bone marrow to make red cells. When copper is low, iron accumulates in the liver. A basic multivitamin with minerals generally provides adequate amounts of copper and other minerals, but some minerals deserve further explanation.

Selenium

Selenium is a trace mineral that is necessary for various metabolic and antioxidant processes. However, excessive selenium intake can be toxic. Selenium is involved in antioxidant reactions to protect DNA from damage. It also produces T-cells, which destroy cells damaged by viruses or bacteria or that have become cancerous. Selenium also supports thyroid hormone production, like T3.

Selenium deficiency increases the risk of viral infections. Supplementation of selenium helps prevent people infected with the hepatitis B and C virus from developing liver cancer.

Low levels of selenium are associated with a higher risk of lung, stomach, colorectal, and prostate cancer. Selenium and iodine are closely related, and iodine deficiency may worsen hypothyroidism if selenium is supplemented.

Selenium is found in Brazil nuts, shrimp, crabmeat, salmon, pork, chicken, beef, whole grains, garlic, onions, and leeks. A daily dosage of 100 mcg is safe as a supplement.

Plant foods obtain selenium from the soil, which affects the amount of selenium in animals eating those plants. <u>Protein-rich foods</u> from animals are generally good sources of selenium. Seafood, organ meats, and Brazilian nuts have the highest selenium levels, although Americans obtain most of their selenium from everyday staples, like breads, cereals, poultry, red meat, and eggs.

Calcium

Calcium is an essential mineral involved in many functions of all cells. It helps to keep bones strong and teeth healthy and is crucial for muscle and nerve function, heart function, and blood clotting. Calcium from vegetable sources is better, as calcium from stones or mineral sources is responsible for plaque formation and stones. Calcium intake protects against lead toxicity by decreasing lead absorption in water or foods. A diet rich in fruits, vegetables, poultry, and milk products usually provides enough calcium for the average person. Pregnant women, however, should get enough calcium to reduce preeclampsia risk and help their baby's bones develop correctly. If you take calcium supplements, I recommend no more than 500 mg a day.

Too much calcium in the diet or through supplements may impair the absorption of other essential minerals and can even be harmful. It can cause kidney stones and may contribute to hardening of the arteries. For example, if you take calcium to combat osteoporosis, you must also take vitamins D and K, magnesium, iron, and zinc. Combined preparations of these minerals are available. Calcium alone without vitamin D is not effective in preventing osteoporosis. I recommend taking magnesium in the evening or before bed at night.

Chromium

This mineral plays a role in regulating blood sugar levels. You only need traces of this mineral. Chromium exists in two forms: trivalent form, which is found in food and is necessary for biological functions, and hexavalent, which is an industrial form that is toxic if consumed. The only type of chromium that is safe is the one found in natural foods and supplements. You should never try the industrial form. Vitamin C and some B vitamins are needed to absorb chromium in the gut. This combination is another reason to use a daily multivitamin with minerals. Research suggests that chromium helps decrease binge eating and weight gain. Chromium allows insulin to enter the cells, making them more sensitive to insulin and helping maintain good blood sugar levels. Chromium also helps to lower triglycerides and raise good cholesterol or HDL in those taking beta-blockers. Chromium is helpful to control and improve acne and insulin resistance.

Brewer's yeast is a good source of biologically active chromium and more effective than chromium supplements. Meat, eggs, tomatoes, green beans, nuts, whole grains, and meats are good sources of chromium.

Consuming highly refined and processed foods increases chromium excretion. People with inflammatory bowel disease may be low in chromium.

Consuming highly refined and processed foods increases chromium excretion. People with inflammatory bowel disease may be low in chromium.

Chromium picolinate is the most common form of supplementation, and a daily dose of 120 mcg a day is sufficient for most people. Prediabetics; type 2 diabetics; people with absorption problems, acne, low HDL, or high triglycerides; those taking beta-blockers; and many athletes may have higher requirements, with a target dosage of 400 mcg daily. Chromium picolinate combined with vitamin C and 2 mg of biotin daily improved blood glucose and cholesterol levels in type 2 diabetics and prediabetics.

Iodine

Iodine is a mineral essential for the production of thyroid hormones. Without iodine, a person develops hypothyroidism. People who are deficient in thyroid hormone gain weight, become obese and feel tired. They also may have dry skin, muscle cramps, fatigue, intolerance to cold, puffy eyes, constipation, poor memory, and slow thinking. Diets that exclude iodine salt, seafood, and dairy products lead to lower levels of iodine.

Vegans are at risk of developing iodine deficiency. The Oxford Vegetarian Study found similar results with vegans in the United Kingdom. This deficiency may be because of the marginal iodine intake and the higher intake of goitrogenic vegetables. Most cruciferous vegetables are goitrogenic. They include arugula, bok choy, broccoli, Brussels sprouts, cabbage, cauliflower, kale, collard greens, mustard greens, turnips, and watercress. The goitrogenic effect in these vegetables has no impact if the diet contains significant iodine levels.

Another factor to consider is using chemicals like bromide to purify whirlpools and as a pesticide in fruits like strawberries. Bromide displaces iodine from its receptors, which leads to iodine deficiencies. Baked foods contain potassium bromide, and some sodas have brominated vegetable oils. Other chemicals that may affect the levels of iodine and the production of thyroid hormones are perchlorate, thiocyanate, nitrate, and phthalate. In a controlled antenatal thyroid study in the United Kingdom and Turin, Italy, from 2002 to 2006, 21,846 women who were less than sixteen weeks pregnant were tested. Perchlorate was present in all the women, and their iodine levels were low. Women with high perchlorate levels have a 300 percent increase in odds of having babies with low IQ at three years of age. Since perchlorate is present in the mammary glands, it can potentially decrease iodine levels in their babies.

The daily recommended iodine intake is 150 mcg for men and women. These requirements are higher during pregnancy and breastfeeding. The American Thyroid Association and the Endocrine Society recommend a multivitamin-mineral supplement containing 150 mcg of potassium iodide/iodine daily. This dosage should continue during breastfeeding to ensure the iodine passes from the breast milk to the baby.

During pregnancy, the thyroid hormone is essential for developing the baby's nerves and brain. Iodine deficiency during pregnancy is associated with high incidences of attention deficit disorder (ADHD), lower IQ, and mental retardation. The World Health Organization (WHO) identifies iodine deficiency as the leading cause of cognitive impairment in children, affecting over 2.3 billion people worldwide.

Fortunately, iodine is present in iodized salt. Sea salt doesn't contain enough iodine. It would help if you bought iodized table salt or iodized sea salt. You may want to eat seaweed, which contains iodine. Remember that the salt in fast foods is not iodized and does not help produce thyroid hormones. When exposed to the air, salt left in a shaker for over four weeks loses 40 percent of its iodine. Loss of iodine may result in iodine deficiency and hypothyroidism. People on low-salt diets do not get an adequate amount of iodine and will develop hypothyroidism. I recommend they take a multivitamin with minerals that contains 150 mcg of iodine or add seaweed to their diets.

Low iron levels can exacerbate low levels of iodine. This deficiency is especially true for pregnant women. Therefore, pregnant women should take a multivitamin that contains at least 150 mcg of iodine and iron. Pregnant and lactating women should take from 220 to 290 mcg daily. Both iron and iodine are essential in the process of making the thyroid hormone. In the United States, roughly 99 percent of processed foods do not contain iodine. People on low-salt diets or diuretics suffer from iodine deficiencies. Hispanic and black women often have the highest deficits of iron and iodine and could have children with mental deficiencies. This deficiency is preventable by taking vitamins that contain iodine and iron during pregnancy and breastfeeding.

Good sources of iodine are fish, shellfish, eggs, and seaweed. Seaweed has the highest levels of highly bioavailable iodine and is the top food source. Iodized table salt loses iodine within two months of opening the package. Due to its excellent stability, the WHO recommends ionization with potassium iodate, particularly in humid and tropical areas.

Any diet deficient in iron, iodine, zinc, and magnesium most likely will lead to health problems. Iron is part of the thyroid peroxidase enzyme necessary to make thyroid hormones. Hair loss, or alopecia areata, may be one early sign of iodine deficiency. Iron and iodine are required to provide strength to the hair. If you are losing hair, gaining weight, experiencing an enlarged thyroid gland, or suspect you are at a higher risk of having children with mental retardation, ask your doctor to run blood tests to check for deficiencies in T3, T4, T7, TSH, serum ferritin levels, TBIC (total iron-binding capacity), zinc, and magnesium.

Since my prescription for healthy living is to help you live longer and reach your final destination in optimal health, you should have these tests as part of a yearly physical as you age. If you begin to develop any of the symptoms noted above, ask your doctor or order the test from labs that do not require a doctor's order and are available in the resources section.

People at risk for iodine deficiency include those who do not use iodized salt or supplements containing iodine, pregnant women, vegans who do not eat any animal foods, and those living in areas with low levels of iodine in the soil (e.g., mountainous regions).

High iodine intakes are usually well-tolerated in most healthy people and do not cause problems in countries such as Japan and Korea that eat iodine-rich seaweed regularly. However, some people with autoimmune thyroid disease or who have a history of chronic iodine deficiency can be sensitive to receiving extra iodine, inducing conditions of iodine deficiency like hypothyroidism and goiter. [2,4] Excess iodine can also lead to too much thyroid hormone production, causing hyperthyroidism; signs of this condition are an increased metabolism that promotes weight loss, fast or irregular heartbeat, hand tremors, irritability, fatigue, and sweatiness. Sometimes, a slight increase in dietary iodine above the RDA can cause iodine-induced hyperthyroidism in sensitive individuals.

Some epidemiologic studies have shown that high seaweed intakes are associated with an increased risk of certain types of thyroid cancer, particularly in postmenopausal women, but the exact mechanism is unclear.

Excess iodine intake may come from high-dose supplements or overeating certain seaweeds and salts containing iodine. Severe iodine poisoning is rare, but symptoms include fever, stomach pain, nausea, vomiting, a burning sensation in the mouth, throat, and stomach, and even coma. Children, infants, older adults, and those with existing thyroid disease are particularly vulnerable to iodine toxicity and iodine-induced hypothyroidism and hyperthyroidism.

For your information:

- In the US, people obtain most of their dietary iodine from iodized salt and milk.
- Iodine supplements can interact with certain blood pressure medications and diuretics, including lisinopril, spironolactone, and amiloride, causing a dangerous buildup of potassium in the blood, a condition known as hyperkalemia.
- Iodine is also an ingredient in contrast agents that a person may take before having an X-ray or computed tomography (CT) scan.

Iron

Iron is a mineral that, according to WHO, is the most deficient nutrient in the world. Iron is available in both animal and plant foods. This deficiency is staggering in developing nations and is usually associated with parasitic infections, malaria, and T.BT.B. Iron deficiency anemia contributes to about 20 percent of all maternal deaths in the world. Anemia in the mother contributes to premature and low birth weight, which will impair the child's cognitive and behavioral development. I believe vitamins with iron and minerals must be accessible to all women worldwide during pregnancy and lactation. Taking too much iron for too long may be dangerous. If a person has no anemia and iron levels are normal, there is no need for additional iron. Iron can be toxic when taken in excess. Iron can accumulate in all organs, causing damage to the liver, pancreas, heart, and brain. The only solution for too much iron in the body is to donate blood regularly and avoid taking additional iron. It is always wise to use iron only under the direction of a doctor.

Iron deficiency develops from low dietary intake, poor absorption, or blood loss. In my practice, I find people who complain of easy fatigue or weakness and dizziness to sometimes be anemic. Usually, the first question is why this is happening. In women, excessive loss of blood during menstruation or gastrointestinal bleeding by stomach ulcers or hemorrhoids may be the cause. A complete blood test and differential CBC are essential tests. Other causes may be a diet deficient in iron or poor iron absorption. Deficiencies in vitamin B12 or folic acid may also cause anemia. It is crucial to see a doctor if you are anemic or losing too much blood.

Iron is necessary to make hemoglobin, the protein in red cells that carries oxygen to the tissues. More than 60 percent of our iron is in hemoglobin. Iron is also present in myoglobin, a protein in the muscles that provide sufficient oxygen to hardworking muscles.

When iron is low, hemoglobin levels drop, as does tissue oxygen. With less oxygen, the tissues can't perform their metabolic functions and produce energy. Without enough oxygen, the muscles can't do their jobs, and a person feels weak. The brain is also affected. A lack of oxygen to the brain causes dizziness and a lack of attention and concentration.

Anemic children are unable to concentrate and learn anything in school. Some doctors and counselors recommend psychostimulants to children to improve their concentration when the real problem is anemia and treatment of nutritional deficiencies, including iron. Parents must request a CBC, a complete dietary assessment, and iron levels before considering psychostimulants.

The daily recommended allowance of iron is 8 mg for men and 18 mg for women aged nineteen to fifty. After menopause, the requirement drops to 8 mg for women. During pregnancy, the requirement is 27 mg per day and 9 mg during breastfeeding.

Vegetarians should double these minimum requirements.

Food has two forms of iron—the heme and the nonheme. Meat contains both forms, while plants contain only the nonheme iron.

We absorb only 18 percent of the heme iron and 10 percent of the nonheme. This nonheme could decrease to 2 percent in a vegetarian, mainly eating beans, rice, grains, soybeans, and lentils due to a compound called phytic acid that reduces iron absorption.

The absorption is also increased by legumes with vitamin C. Another way to increase the absorption of nonheme iron is to add chili peppers, which are a great vitamin C. Eat shellfish and nuts; dried foods and fortified foods are also good sources of iron, as cooked spinach is a good source of iron.

In the US, 7 percent of children aged one to five are iron deficient, with higher rates among Mexican Americans. In America, 10 percent of women between 12 and 49 years of age are iron deficient. This number is 12 percent for Latinas and 16 percent for black women. These numbers are even higher in pregnant women, and these deficiencies may affect children's cognitive development.

Magnesium

Magnesium is an essential mineral that aids the proper function of calcium and the activity of vitamin D, by converting vitamin D into its active form. Magnesium is involved in the metabolism of carbohydrates and fats and the production of DNA, RNA, and many proteins. This mineral is involved in nerve and muscle activity, helping to maintain a healthy heart rhythm.

Magnesium is necessary for the synthesis of Glutathione, which is one of the most essential antioxidants. It also helps to lower blood pressure by relaxing the blood vessels. Using magnesium as a supplement in treating hypertension is a good idea. In pregnant women with preeclampsia, magnesium helps to lower blood pressure, reducing the risks of seizures or maternal death. Magnesium prevents sudden cardiac death, which is responsible for more than fifty percent of cardiac deaths. Studies have shown that people with low magnesium levels (less than 1.77 mg/dL) have a higher risk of atrial fibrillation. Additionally, a Japanese study showed that people with a higher intake of magnesium have a lower risk of developing a stroke or heart failure.

Magnesium helps in maintaining normal blood sugar levels, preventing diabetes. Studies have shown that increasing magnesium intake may lower the risk of diabetes by 22 percent. When blood sugar rises, magnesium is lost through urine, causing people with diabetes to suffer from a magnesium deficiency. Scientific studies suggest that magnesium supplementation is protective and helps decrease inflammation.

Magnesium increases enzyme activity that helps your body use vitamin D and regulates calcium. All enzymes that metabolize vitamin D require magnesium to work. As with vitamin D and K2, a magnesium deficiency is present in many people. You may exacerbate the situation if you are low in magnesium and take supplemental calcium. If you take a calcium supplement, you should include magnesium, vitamin D, and K2. Magnesium helps to relax muscles, prevents cramps, and helps people to relax and sleep. Low levels of magnesium reduce serotonin levels, which leads to depression. People with anxiety and depression feel better with magnesium supplementation.

Magnesium has many benefits. For example, several studies show that it can be more effective than ibuprofen and naproxen in treating migraines. Magnesium with vitamin B6 helps to reduce menstrual cramps, anxiety, and irritability. It also decreases breast tenderness, menstrual weight gain, and pain. Taking magnesium at night helps to relieve muscle cramps, promoting a good restful sleep. Magnesium also plays a role in elevating levels of good HDL or good cholesterol. Intravenous (IV) magnesium is beneficial for patients with severe asthma that does not respond to other medications. I often recommend magnesium to people with insomnia and fibromyalgia.

Dietary sources of magnesium include various vegetables such as spinach, black beans, pumpkin seeds, almonds, cashews, peanut butter, avocados, wheat bread, brown rice, yogurt, salmon, milk, dark chocolate, and sea vegetables. Taking too much calcium and salt causes magnesium loss and low levels. Women on oral contraceptives who have low magnesium levels are at risk of developing blood clots and strokes. Women who suffer from headaches while taking contraceptives should take magnesium supplements.

Among the supplements, magnesium citrate and magnesium threonate are some of the best forms. An optimal dose of magnesium is around 400 mg a day. Too much magnesium citrate can cause diarrhea. Magnesium citrate helps treat constipation. It is available in bottles that look like a soda. Half the bottle is sometimes enough to relieve constipation since it is a good laxative. Magnesium gels and lotions help to relax muscles and reduce muscle cramps. Since magnesium can be absorbed through the skin to some degree, bathing with Epsom salts (magnesium sulfate) helps to relax muscles. Many commercial preparations of calcium, magnesium, and vitamin D in liquid form are beneficial in creating a good balance of these critical minerals and assisting with many bodily functions.

Magnesium helps to increase the production of melatonin. Taking magnesium at night, along with foods rich in melatonin, can help restore normal circadian rhythms. Foods high in melatonin include almonds, spinach, avocados, pineapples, oranges, and bananas. You can prepare a salad using all these foods with salmon every night to help you sleep better. My "Nice Sleep Salad" is a way to help those with sleeping problems to increase their melatonin levels. See Appendix F. Melatonin is a hormone that decreases by 14 percent every decade. It is no wonder that sleeping becomes more challenging as we age!

Zinc and Boron

Zinc and boron are other essential cofactors interacting with vitamin D. Zinc deficiency has also been linked to contributing to Alzheimer's disease. Zinc helps strengthen the immune system, heal wounds, improve skin rashes and problems, decrease prostate inflammation, and enhances the senses of smell and taste. Zinc is involved in the average growth and development of organs and tissues. It is present in shellfish, red meat, poultry, beans, nuts, and whole grains. The body does not store zinc and deficiencies are common in people with inflammation, arthritis, diabetes, and intestinal absorption problems. Pregnant women with zinc deficiencies are at risk of having premature babies, who, in turn, may have abnormal growth and development. Zinc is involved in the expression of many genes and is present in the cell nucleus to repair defective DNA, replication, and transcription. Men need a higher daily requirement of zinc because of the production of testosterone. Zinc concentration is high in the prostate gland, testes, and sperm. When men are deficient in zinc, they may suffer from low testosterone and infertility.

Zinc is essential for maintaining a robust immune system because it activates T lymphocytes, which destroy cells infected with viruses and bacteria or those that have become cancerous. Other white cells like macrophages, neutrophils, and killer cells use zinc to increase their defensive role against infection. When a person has a cold, it is better to use zinc instead of vitamin C, as zinc lozenges can reduce the severity of a cold if taken within twenty-four hours after the onset of symptoms.

Zinc is involved in the production of collagen and the healing of wounds, by activating collagenase, an enzyme involved in the production of collagen. As we age, collagen losses in the dermis, leading to wrinkles. Taking zinc helps to activate collagenase to keep producing collagen, restore the structure of the dermis, and decrease the effects of aging. Zinc also mineralizes bones, making them stronger and less likely to break.

Zinc is a structural component of many antioxidants that help prevent damage by free radicals through oxidative stress. Zinc is in superoxide dismutase, the most potent antioxidant, and a powerful anti-inflammatory. When zinc levels are low, the synthesis of powerful antioxidant enzymes decreases, and the level of oxidative stress increases, exposing the DNA to more damage. Because people with diabetes have higher levels of DNA damage, they may be more susceptible to cancer.

Zinc, when combined with vitamin A, improves our vision by producing a retinal-binding protein, which delivers vitamin A to the retina to improve night vision. When combined with antioxidants, zinc helps to prevent macular degeneration and blindness. Zinc protects red and inflamed gums and prevents canker sores. In 2012, a study published in the Journal of Affective Disorders suggested that zinc supplementation is beneficial in treating depression when combined with antidepressants.

Prolonged intake of higher doses of zinc may affect levels of copper.

Boron is a trace mineral found in many fruits and vegetables. It is essential for bone health because it helps to prevent calcium loss. It also helps to increase the production of sex hormones and build muscles for athletic performance. A daily supplement of 3 mg of born is enough to maintain bone health, and its best sources include apples, broccoli, and root vegetables.

For a better source of vitamins and minerals, the best advice is to take a multivitamin that contains all minerals once a day. I recommend different multivitamins in Appendix A. For specific deficiencies and problems of absorption from the gut, it's better to take the vitamins separately to address the deficiency. Children, pregnant women, vegetarians, and people who drink alcohol are at higher risk of developing mineral deficiencies. A good multivitamin helps to keep our bodies in balance and perfect equilibrium and prevent deficiencies. Vegetarians need additional vitamin B12. People with diabetes need complex B vitamins and some minerals in higher dosages. Chromium picolinate, 500 mg, may help increase insulin sensitivity, lower triglycerides, and raise good cholesterol (HDL).

People taking cholesterol-lowering drugs can benefit by taking CoQ10 and vitamin K2 to prevent plaque formation in the coronary arteries.

Supplements

Many supplements provide nutrients that are unavailable in foods or insufficient in a diet to meet the needs of a growing child or an active adult. Many older people's diets are deficient in many nutrients. Because of chronic inflammation triggered by many senescent cells, there is a deficiency of nutrients to compensate for many chemical processes. Hormone deficiencies are an example. Women, as they reach menopause, should compensate for deficiencies of estrogens and testosterone. Something similar for men who begin to experience a decrease in their libido and eréctil dysfunction. Hormone replacement is a way to supplement these deficits to keep the hormonal system in equilibrium. Many supplements support many other biochemical functions, the immune system and inflammation reduction. Below, I am listing some of the supplements I consider more beneficial. I divide them into supplements to fight inflammation, the common denominator of many degenerative and autoimmune diseases, and supplements to support stem cells and cell rejuvenation. I also recommend supplements like Quercetin, which helps to eliminate senescent cells and is known as senolytics (see ahead).

Anti-inflammatory Supplements

Turmeric (Curcumin)

Turmeric is one of the best anti-inflammatory supplements with analgesic qualities. My wife has been using this supplement for over twenty years, and I attribute her youth and good health to its benefits. My wife had arthritis in both hands, which didn't respond to most of the NSAIDs available in the market. She had some success with injections of steroids temporarily. Rather than using chemotherapy and more potent agents that compromise the immune system, she began to take Turmeric in combination with other supplements that have anti-inflammatory properties.

Omega-3 provides anti-inflammatory properties that enhance the effects of Turmeric. In addition, she takes Glucosamine with MSM, Boswellia, and Sam-e, which is an excellent analgesic. With such a combination, she could arrest the inflammation of the joints of her hands. I tried this combination with other patients are seen with similar success. The advantage of these supplements is that they don't have the side effects many patients experience with NSAIDs. Gastric problems like gastritis, ulcers, and stomach pain limit the use of NSAIDs. This combination controls chronic inflammation from other sources and prevents damage to these organs. I feel that by controlling chronic inflammation, a person slows the appearance of wrinkles, arthritis, and a leaky gut. I also think that this anti-inflammatory regimen slows down aging. My wife is proof of this statement. She looks 20 to 30 years younger than her chronological age.

I recommend a dose of 500 mg twice a day to be effective. Turmeric makes people sleepy a few hours after intake. I recommend that you take a small dose in the morning of 125 mg and 750 mg at night. Turmeric can also help you sleep better if you have insomnia or sleep problems.

Researchers found that Turmeric suppresses the release of inflammatory mediators like TNF. Sixteen randomized controlled trials of various Turmeric formulations for knee osteoarthritis, for sixteen weeks, demonstrated a significant reduction of knee pain compared with NSAIDs with a better safety profile.

MSM (Methylsulfonylmethane)

MSM is an abbreviation for **methylsulfonylmethane**, a chemical found naturally in plants and animals. This organic compound, combined with glucosamine hydrochloride and chondroitin sulfate, is a potent anti-inflammation agent. This combination is excellent for treating osteoarthritis, rheumatoid arthritis, tendonitis, and tenosynovitis. Some people use MSM to treat gastrointestinal disorders like constipation, hemorrhoids, diverticulosis rhinitis, seasonal allergies, cough, and respiratory problems.

MSM is essential for supporting many different functions in the body. It is vital for supporting proper cell structure and reversing damage by free radicals to cells. MSM also supports the immune system and the body's ability to repair connective tissue.

Dosages of 1.125 mg three times daily relieve pain and improve joint function. Some studies using 3 grams twice daily have shown significant pain relief compared to a placebo.

Additionally, many skin creams contain MSM, which promises to reduce the appearance of wrinkles when applied topically. Researchers set out to determine if oral supplementation of MSM would produce the same anti-aging result.

Participants took 3 grams of MSM per day for 16 weeks. The photographic analysis showed that the treatment group saw significant improvement in the appearance of crow's feet and overall facial wrinkling.

Omega-3

Omega-3, found in fish oil, helps reduce inflammation by increasing anti-inflammatory mediators that help regulate inflammation.

A review of 73 studies published in *International Immunopharmacology* found that adults who take an omega-3 fatty acid supplement, including fish oil, improved markers of inflammation in various health conditions such as cancer, kidney diseases, and diabetes. Additionally, omega-3 supplementation has shown promise regarding brain health, particularly memory, cognition, and blood flow to the brain. My wife and I take omega-3 every day. We take a teaspoon of omega-3 liquid in our smoothies every day.

N-acetyl cysteine and Glutathione

<u>N-acetyl cysteine (NAC)</u> is a compound made from one of the building blocks of protein, known as the amino acid L-cysteine, with antioxidant functions. NAC's primary role in the body is to act as a precursor to Glutathione, one of the body's most powerful antioxidant that is known to combat oxidative stress.

When Glutathione decreases, researchers believe the body might be more susceptible to chronic inflammation and disease progression. I recommend NAC as a precursor to Glutathione for its beneficial effects.

NAD+ and NMN

NAD+ and its precursor NMN Nicotinamide mononucleotide) are small-chain amino acid peptides that help activate vital cellular function in the body. Some studies suggest it helps improve memory and the progression of Alzheimer's. Other benefits include DNA repair, regulation of circadian rhythm, and stem cell rejuvenation. Both are available as supplements.

I recommend boosting your NAD+ levels by taking NMN daily as an oral supplement. One to two capsules of 500 mg a day, preferably in the morning with breakfast.

As you age, your levels of NAD+ decline. Restoring your NDA+ levels with the NMN precursor is the best way to go. These chemicals help to prevent muscle wasting, and many of the chronic effects of aging. The pro-longevity effects are supported by growing scientific evidence. David Sinclair, a Harvard scientist, says that we lose NAD+ as we age resulting in a decline of sirtuin activity, which is the primary reason our bodies develop diseases when we are old and not when we are young. He believes that increasing the levels of NAD+ reverses the aging process.

In addition to NMN, polyphenols from a plant-based diet, exercise, and caloric restriction, the NAD+ levels could increase and activate sirtuins.

Sirtuins protect against diabetes and fatty liver by improving insulin secretion from the pancreas, promoting fat metabolism and increasing liver glucose production. Sirtuins protect against muscle wasting, neurodegenerative diseases and fat gain. Several studies suggest that by increasing DNA+ the body can fight viruses like COVID-19 and the cytokine storm associated with COVID death. Since older people have lower levels of NAD+, they are more susceptible to viral infections like COVID-19 and many other viruses.

DNA+ protects the mitochondria and the output of energy. Aging and fat rich diets reduce the levels of DNA+. A plant-based diet low in saturated fats combined with exercise prolongs lifespan and improves cardiac function, protects the brain from neurodegeneration and memory loss.

Bromelain

Bromelain is an enzyme naturally found in the fruit and stems of pineapple.

It appears to have many health benefits, including helping with inflammation and pain.

In a study of 103 people with osteoarthritis (OA), 52 received a bromelain-containing mixture, and 51 received NSAIDs. Bromelain was an effective and safe alternative to NSAIDs in the treatment of painful episodes of OA of the knee.

Green tea

Green tea is an excellent anti-aging supplement that offers various benefits. It is known for its anti-inflammatory, antioxidant, anti-cancer, and neuroprotective properties. Compared to black tea, green tea is a healthier option due to the way it is processed. While black tea leaves can oxidize and turn darker, green tea leaves are protected from air exposure, resulting in a lighter color and a different nutrient profile. Both black and green tea contain flavonoids, which are antioxidants. However, green tea has significantly higher essential flavonoids like EGCG (Epigallocathechin-3-gallate), a potent DNA methylation adaptogen. Green tea is also lower in caffeine and less dehydrating than black tea. Matcha is a powerful form of green tea that you can enjoy as a delicious Matcha latte.

Green tea positively affects telomeres, increasing telomerase activity to lengthen telomeres. As recommended in my DRESS-SS prescription, a plant-based diet and a wellness lifestyle appear to do the same. Dr. Ornish's studies demonstrated that a plant-based diet rich in fiber and lifestyle changes enlongated telomeres, a finding echoed by Nobel Prize of Medicine winner Elizabeth Blackburn in her book *"The Telomere Effect."*

What is interesting is the influence of the epigenome in increasing the telomere length with lifestyle changes.

Resveratrol

Resveratrol is a natural polyphenol detected in more than 70 plant species, especially in grapes' skin and seeds, in discrete amounts in red wines and various human foods. It is a phytoalexin that acts against pathogens, including bacteria and fungi. Numerous studies have demonstrated that resveratrol possesses a very high antioxidant potential as a natural food ingredient. Resveratrol also exhibits antitumor properties, and is considered a potential candidate for preventing and treating several types of cancer. Indeed, resveratrol anti-cancer properties have been confirmed by many in vitro and in vivo studies, which show that resveratrol can inhibit all carcinogenesis stages (e.g., initiation, promotion, and progression). Other bioactive effects, such as anti-inflammatory, anticarcinogenic, cardioprotective, vasorelaxant, phytoestrogens, and neuroprotective, have also been reported. Nonetheless, resveratrol application is still a significant challenge for the pharmaceutical industry due to its poor solubility, bioavailability, and adverse effects.

I take 500mg of resveratrol every morning. I recommend this dosage. If resveratrol is part of an anti-cancer regimen, you should consult your oncologist.

Quercetin

Quercetin is a natural plant-derived polyphenol with anti-inflammatory, antioxidant, and anti-aging properties. It has been shown to reduce periodontal bone loss and prevents disease progression in animal models of experimental periodontal disease. Quercetin might facilitate periodontal tissue hemostasis by reducing senescent cells, decreasing oxidative stress via SIRT1-induced autophagy, limiting inflammation, and fostering an oral bacterial microenvironment of symbiotic microbiota associated with oral health. Quercetin is a safe, natural compound that is very useful in treating periodontitis, particularly in older adults who do not need antibiotics.

The flavonoid quercetin has been part of the human diet for centuries, and is found in various fruits (e.g., apples, cranberries, and grapes) and vegetables (e.g., onion, capers, and traditional herbs). Quercetin acts as a senolytic agent byactivating mechanisms that eliminate the accumulation of senescent cells. It triggers apoptosis through a mitochondrial pathway that activates caspase-3 and caspase-9 by releasing cytochrome C.

Furthermore, Quercetin suppresses oral bacteria by damaging the cell envelope, refraining bacterial adhesion, blocking nucleic acid synthesis, and inhibiting pathogen-related biofilms. Zeng et al. demonstrated that compared to chlorhexidine, quercetin effectively reduced biofilm dry weight, total protein content, and the number of viable cells in *Streptococcus mutans biofilms.*

Quercetin's anti-inflammatory properties comes from blocking TNF-α-mediated inflammation in macrophage cells and inhibiting cyclooxygenase and lipoxygenase pathways.

Quercetin is a substance with distinctive biological activities that can treat cardiovascular and degenerative neuronal diseases. It acts as a potent antioxidant by scavenging reactive oxygen species, inhibiting lipid peroxidation, and increasing the activity of antioxidant enzymes. The reduction in oxidative stress in the brain supports protection against neurodegenerative diseases. Additionally, Quercetin inhibits the activation of microglial cells and reduces the production of pro-inflammatory cytokines, thereby reducing inflammation in the brain and adding to the neuroprotective effects. Additionally, quercetin has beneficial effects on blood pressure by improving endothelial function, potentially rendering the endothelium less vulnerable to injury and senescence. Its senolytic impact stimulates autophagy of endothelial cells, contributing to cardiovascular health.

Quercetin is available as a supplement alone or combined with bromelain and Turmeric in vegetarian capsules of 500 mg. It can be taken one or two times a day, depending on the severity of periodontitis or the presence of senescent cells. You may need a lower dosage of fruits and vegetables rich in Quercetin.

Quercetin helps in preventing periodontal disease and bone loss.

Periodontal disease progresses by deregulated inflammation and dysbiotic microbiota. Hence, both clinical conditions respond to treatment by the polyphenol quercetin. Mooney et al. reported that Quercetin enables sustained periodontal tissue homeostasis in mice and moderates the disease by modulating the inflammatory response and the oral microbial composition. In human macrophage-like cells exposed to lipopolysaccharide and periodontal bacteria, Quercetin reduced cytokine production through its effect on NF-κB signaling.

Research data shows that quercetin supplementation might facilitate periodontal tissue hemostasis by reducing senescent cells, limiting inflammation, and fostering an oral bacterial microenvironment of symbiotic microbiota associated with oral health. Hence, Quercetin could be effective in treating and preventing periodontitis.

Research studies show less alveolar bone loss than control animals without quercetin administration. A meta-analysis resulted in a significant beneficial effect of Quercetin in preventing periodontal disease.

Quercetin is a crystalline yellowish substance with a bitter flavor. High levels of quercetin are available in fruits and vegetables like apples, cranberries, grapes, onions, and capers. Depending on food intake and consumption of fruits and vegetables, the dietary intake of Quercetin ranges from 50 to 800 mg per day.

The flavonoid quercetin has a high antioxidant capacity and is an effective free radical scavenger. In vivo, quercetin's antioxidant mechanism is due to its effects on Glutathione, signal transduction pathways, and reactive oxygen species. It can remove reactive oxygen species and reduce oxidative damage caused by ultraviolet radiation B (UVB) in the skin.

Quercetin showed long-lasting and robust anti-inflammatory properties in many tissues. Pro-apoptotic autophagy via the SIRT1/AMPK signaling pathway occurs by Quercetin in non-small-cell cancer cell lines in vitro.

Quercetin ameliorated cigarette smoke-related periodontal tissue destruction in mice by reducing oxidative stress damage and autophagy dysfunction.

Quercetin downregulated overall DNA methylation levels in a dose and time-dependent way. Combined with Quercetin, Dasatinib diminished senescent cell burden and reduced pro-inflammatory cytokine secretion in human adipose tissue. Quercetin, again with additional dasatinib, was shown to clear senescent cells in an atrial fibrillation mouse model and ameliorate cardiac function. Modulating cell senescence might provide a basis for new therapeutic approaches to atrial fibrillation.

Senescent cells play a role in the pathogenesis of periodontitis and contribute to the development of peri-implantitis. Yang et al. showed that senescent cells exacerbate peri-implantitis in animals receiving dental implants. The peri-implantitis rat model treated with senolytics (dasatinib and quercetin) reduced implant loss by preventing senescence-related mechanisms. In bone augmentation, ß-tricalcium phosphate granules induced senescence-like cells, after administering a senolytic combination of dasatinib. It enhances the bone-forming capability of β-tricalcium phosphate. Additionally, a 4% quercetin/polycaprolactone fibrous membrane showed enhanced periodontal bone regeneration in an in vivo rat model compared to an unloaded membrane.

Immunosenescence is a progressive immune system modification that increases susceptibility to infections, cancer, and autoimmune manifestations. In periodontal disease, alterations in the function of local cells of the periodontium contribute to the phenomenon known as "inflammaging". Pathophysiologic changes associated with aging aggravate periodontal disease and are likely responsible for the higher incidence of periodontal disease in older people. Treatment of this senescent phenotype might be therapeutically beneficial and could ameliorate periodontal disease. Bertolini et al. highlighted periodontal disease as a chronic inflammatory condition linked to aging. They proposed that periodontal disease might be an effective geroscience model to study mechanisms of age-related inflammatory dysregulation. Age-related changes in immune cells lead to less effective clearance of microbial pathogens and increased pro-inflammatory cytokine secretion. Quercetin, with its senolytic properties, eliminate senescent cells and contribute to the restoration of a more stable periodontal situation.

Quercetin and resveratrol have been shown to reduce the inflammatory process in apical periodontitis, particularly in cases of periapical bone resorption. These compounds increased osteoprotegerin Il-10 and decreased tartrate-resistant acid phosphatase expression compared to the control. Research by Ge et al. demonstrated that Quercetin increased the number of M2 macrophages, IL-10, and osteoprotegerin and reduced RANKL. Quercetin inhibited the growth of microbial pathogens like Staphylococcus aureus, Pseudomonas aeruginosa, and Escherichia coli. Quercetin inhibited the formation of S. aureus biofilms. It interfered with pathways involved in bacterial quorum sensing, thus preventing bacterial adhesion and biofilm formation. Additionally, Quercetin inhibited biofilm formation, adhesion, and invasion of Candida albicans, reducing inflammation caused by C. albicans and protecting the integrity of the mucosa. In mice studies, Quercetin promoted gut homeostasis by stimulating beneficial bacterial populations like Bifidobacterium sp. and Lactobacillus sp., while inhibiting potentially harmful bacteria such as Enterococcus sp. and Fusobacterium sp.

Quercetin damaged the cell membrane and showed antimicrobial effects against Porphyromonas gingivalis. Additionally, it reduced gingipain expression, hemagglutination, hemolytic activity, and the expression of virulence genes in P. gingivalis, while also inhibiting biofilm formation at subinhibitory concentrations. However, the concentrations used were high and could not be expected at the disease site when applied systemically. A local application of Quercetin may enhance its concentration and boost its antimicrobial effects in the oral cavity.

Quercetin has a generally good safety profile. Quercetin, along with its more soluble derivatives, has received approval from the FDA for human use and is generally considered safe (GRAS). However, studies on chronic toxicity in animals, particularly with high doses of Quercetin, have indicated an increase in nephrotoxic effects, especially in people with kidney disease. Dietary polyphenols like Quercetin might offer various benefits. They are not a panacea but should be part of a well-adjusted diet when reasonably administered. Various foods contain different kinds and amounts of polyphenols, and integrating fruits, vegetables, nuts, and grains into the diet will maximize the benefits of dietary polyphenols. I recommend moderate intake of polyphenols like Quercetin, as disproportionate consumption may not be beneficial and lead to adverse effects.

Supplements for Cell Rejuvenation

A diet rich in fruits and vegetables such as kale, blueberries, ginger, nuts, broccoli, shiitake mushrooms, spirulina, raspberries, and acai berries promotes cell and stem cell rejuvenation. These foods are rich in antioxidants, vitamins, minerals, and phytochemicals that help protect and repair cells.

Fish oil: This supplement contains omega-3 and omega-6 fatty acids in the right proportion, 4:1, which supports membrane formation and protection. Fish oil also helps reduce inflammation and support cell membrane function.

Other promising supplements that may support cell regeneration and overall health:

Vitamins A, C, and E:

- **Vitamin A**: Essential for cell regeneration, it plays a key role in creating new cells.
- **Vitamin C**: Improves circulation and skin health, aiding in cell regeneration.
- **Vitamin E: Protects against cellular damage and supports overall longevity.**
- **EGCG (Epigallocatechin Gallate): Found in green tea, EGCG restores mitochondrial function, induces autophagy (cellular material removal), and may protect against** skin aging.
- **Curcumin (from Turmeric)**: Activates proteins that delay cellular senescence, combat cellular damage, and may increase lifespan.

CHAPTER 5

Longevity and Aging

Why do we age? How can you live longer by eating the right foods?

Eos asked Zeus to grant Tithonus eternal life, and the god consented and granted her wish. But Eos forgot to ask for eternal youth, so her husband grew old and withered. When she returned to ask for eternal youth, it was too late.

According to the Homeric *Hymn to Aphrodite.*

Many people dread getting old. They see aging as a time of decay, pain, and suffering. We cannot deny such reality.

In this chapter, I will explore the concept of longevity and how dietary choices can impact our aging process.

Historically, we live longer than our ancestors hundreds of years ago. We should be optimistic. If we direct our thoughts to make that possible, we can remain healthier, young, and full of physical and mental vitality.

This Homeric poem illustrates our dilemma. What is the best choice between two equal and desirable alternatives? Why not live longer and remain healthier until our last breath?

But what is the best choice between living longer or eternal health? Living longer without lasting health is not a good choice, as was the case with Tithonus in the Greek legend.

Lasting health is probably better so we can live longer because living longer without health is not a good alternative.

The myth highlights the undesirable consequences of longevity without vitality- a scenario that modern science seeks to prevent.

Our quest for better health continues. We are living longer than our ancestors did over 100 years ago. We enjoy better health and longevity because of our knowledge about nutritional research, better nutrition, antibiotics, medical technological advances, improvements in public health, diagnosis, and treatments.

The good news is that even more significant medical advances, particularly in cellular biology and genetics, are on the horizon. These breakthroughs hold the potential to improve our health span and treat and cure human diseases through cellular rejuvenation, epigenetic reprogramming, and organ regeneration. The Yamanaka factors, discovered by a Nobel Prize winner, Dr. Yamanaka, have shown the ability to turn back time and restore cells to a youthful state, maintaining their identity and function. By reversing disease and preventing mitochondrial damage by free radicals, scientists may one day eliminate the chronic degenerative diseases that make us age faster than we want. Future generations may not wither as Tithonus did. Science may grant us the wish of lasting life, and possibly even eternal youth. Believe it or not, we have ways to start this process of eternal youth. Restricting methionine, an amino acid in animal protein, helps prolong life.

How long can humans live, and why do we age?

Humans today live longer than in our evolutionary past, but we still experience aging and physical decline at a rate of 1% per year after age 30. Research shows that limiting calorie intake and reducing exposure to free radicals can slow aging. Free radicals come from the metabolism of sugars and proteins in the mitochondria and can attach to biomolecules such as DNA, lipids, and proteins, causing damage.

Some scientists believe aging is biologically programmed, while others argue that it results from environmental and dietary factors, particularly mitochondrial damage. More than three hundred theories of aging have been proposed. In 1956, the free radical theory of aging was proposed because of the parallel between DNA damage caused by radiation exposure and early manifestations of aging. Over time, the realization that the mitochondria were the primary source of cellular free radical formation evolved into what today is known as the mitochondrial theory.

The mitochondrial theory suggests that animals with lower mitochondrial free radical production tend to live longer.

The mitochondria of long-lived species confirm this theory. These animals leak fewer electrons, which correlates with less mitochondrial and DNA oxidative damage.

Another finding has been how methionine content is linked to maximum life span. The lower the methionine intake, the longer the longevity. Methionine is the amino acid most susceptible to oxidation in the mitochondria. High methionine levels don't just make you vulnerable to oxidative stress, though- they actively cause it. In laboratory experiments, researchers decreased the intake of proteins in rodents, decreasing by 40 percent the production of free radicals. Researchers found that the benefits of protein restrictions on mitochondrial function were due to the drop of one single amino acid, methionine. Restricting methionine for just seven weeks halted the leakage of electrons and DNA damage in rodents, reducing methionine intake also reduces aging and related diseases, extending lifespan. There are many ways to prolong life, but methionine restriction alone accounts for 50 percent of the life extension attributed to full dietary restriction.

There are three ways to lower methionine intake. One approach is to decrease protein intake. However, this method will leave us hungry. Another way is to reduce the intake of protein in our diets. A third way is to substitute animal protein for plant-based protein. Longevity researchers have found that restricting methionine from animal sources offers numerous benefits. Data showing legume consumption may be the best survival predictor in older people worldwide, the cornerstone of longevity in the Blue Zone diets. Plant-based diets make methionine restriction possible as a lifespan extension strategy.

Foods with high methionine content include fish, poultry, eggs, red meat, and dairy from animal sources. In contrast, plant foods contain ten times less methionine. Beans have ten times less methionine than fish and poultry, nuts have twenty times less, and vegetables have minimal amounts. This higher content of methionine in animal foods is a good reason to limit the intake of animal foods, as it limits our health span and longevity.

Vegans consume 47 percent less methionine than meat eaters. They are generally 40 pounds lighter than people on regular diets. Vegetarians consume dairy and other foods with a higher content of methionine. They consume 36 percent less methionine. Vegans, due to their plant-based diets appear to be healthier than both vegetarians and those on conventional diets. The reason is a plant-based diet. Since vitamin B12 deficiency may be present in a vegan diet, I recommend taking this vitamin as a supplement or consuming fish like wild salmon once a week.

As previously mentioned, individuals who practice calorie restriction through intermittent fasting and consume plant-based foods produce fewer free radicals and appear biologically younger than those of the same chronological age.

People are increasingly exploring ways to modify genetic control and reduce exposure to harmful elements through diets and lifestyle changes to delay aging. Research demonstrates that the epigenome plays a vital role in the expression of genes. By limiting the expression of genes that predispose to diabetes, cancer, and other illnesses, an individual could prevent the development of a deadly disease. Turning off this gene provides the basis for a longer health span and lifespan. Turning genes on allows the expression of favorable genes. My DRESS-SS prescription, initially described in my first book, provides a method to influence our genetic code by controlling the epigenome.

Are Branched-Chain Amino Acids (BCAAs) Suitable for Your Health?

Three amino acids, known as BCAAs, affect health and longevity besides methionine.

They are isoleucine, leucine, and valine. These are commonly found in supplements for athletes to increase muscle mass. However,

Dr. Greger, in his book *"How Not to Age,"* reports that, in twenty-five diet mega studies, health and longevity negatively correlated with higher levels of BCAA in the blood. People with lower BCAA levels have healthier and longer lives. In animal studies, BCAA shortens mouse lifespan, while BCAA restriction increases their lifespan. Researchers conclude that limiting the intake of BCAAs is the key to a long and healthy life. BCAAs are potent activators of mTOR (mechanistic target of rapamycin), a powerful enzyme involved in the aging process.

Reducing mTOR is essential to improve health and lifespan.

In mouse models, mTOR with high BCAAs demonstrated higher cognitive problems. This finding is consistent with people with higher levels of isoleucine to develop Alzheimer's disease

The intake of saturated fats and BCAAs can cause insulin resistance. Reducing BCAAs in obese mice reduces insulin resistance and obesity. Numerous studies have found that BCAAs cause insulin resistance in humans. Increasing BCAAs in the blood is known as the "BCAA signature" and a hallmark of obesity and diabetes. You can do the same by consuming butter to increase insulin resistance within hours or taking a protein shake made of whey rich in BCAAs.

Supplements rich in BCAAs are a multimillion-dollar industry that boosts muscle mass. Although most of these studies are based on animal models, particularly rat studies, only two human studies showed that BCAAs reduce protein synthesis.

BCAAs are abundant in animal products such as meat, poultry, fish, dairy, and eggs. These foods increase insulin resistance. Plant-based foods have the opposite effect. Substituting animal protein for plant-based protein decreases the risk of diabetes by more than 20 percent. More than a dozen randomized controlled trials have shown changing animal protein for plant-based protein significantly improves blood sugar levels. People on plant-based diets usually have lower insulin levels and insulin resistance. For example, adding egg whites to a plant-based diet increases insulin resistance by 60 percent within four days. Insulin resistance increases by 50 percent by adding tuna to mashed potatoes. On the other hand, adding broccoli cuts the insulin response by 40 percent within thirty minutes. These studies demonstrate the differential effect of plant versus animal protein because of the contrasting amino acid profiles. A prevailing belief that consuming more protein is always healthy is misleading. Drs. Valter Longo and Luigi Fontana advise that reducing protein enables one to live longer. As they explain, "Eating more protein than needed will not increase muscle mass but accelerate aging and increase the risk of developing many chronic diseases."

Do We Have Aging Genes?

I searched everywhere for the answer to this question. If we have genes in charge of making people age, it would be a good reason to start a search for the holy grail and the fountain of youth. One day, I found the answer by reading Dr. David Sinclair's book *"Lifespan, Why We Age and Why We Don't Have to."* As we complete our genetic code map, there is something we won't be able to find. We won't be able to find an aging gene, he said.

We have genes that impact the symptoms of aging. Scientists have found longevity genes that help control our defenses against aging. It offers a pathway to slowing aging through natural, pharmaceutical, and technological interventions. However, scientists have not found a singular gene that causes aging. An aging gene is impossible because our genes didn't evolve to cause aging.

So, why do we age?

If we have no aging genes, why do we age?

The answer to this question is not our genes but the factors influencing them. Trauma can kill anyone at any age. Illness due to bacteria, viruses, and cancer can do the same. Still, if damage to the cells is beyond repair or the capability to recover the structure to function is impaired, cells die or become old or "senescent." From birth, we suffer many stressors that affect the systems and health of our cells. But even under stress, our cells have learned to adapt and protect us against significant diseases, including cancer. Our cells have systems to diminish chronic inflammation, which is at the root of many degenerative diseases characteristic of aging. Diabetes, heart disease, Alzheimer's, autoimmune disorders, arthritis, colitis, atherosclerosis, osteoporosis, muscle wasting, macular degeneration, and metabolic disorders accelerate aging.

What, in reality, drives our cells to succumb is the damage done to the driver of our genetic code, not the code itself. Using the analogy, the genome is like a vehicle, while epigenome is the driver, navigating treacherous pathways to stay on the road without accidents and deliver precious cargo to its destination. The complexity of the epigenome's activity over the genome occurs every second, twenty-four hours a day, within the cells. Specialized proteins located near the genes are in charge of this function. The genome is the vehicle and all his parts components that make up the entire structure. Their equivalent in our cells are the chromosomes and all the genes that make our cells. Genes consist of sequences of amino acids bound by chemicals called methyl and acetyls, containing carbon, oxygen, and hydrogen.

Several proteins work as enzymes in our cells to turn on or off our genes. The gene can be activated, turned on, deactivated, or turned off by removing one chemical tag. These mechanisms, more than our genes, are what control our lives. With their skills, the driver determines what kind of ride we will have to reach our destination during our lifetime on this planet. The driver and his epigenetic skills drive people with similar genes in different directions. Brothers or sisters with similar genes behave differently because of their epigenetics.

Identical human twins raised separately or that have different lifestyles age differently. Lifespan and health may be affected by exposure to cigarette smoke, toxic substances, and unhealthy lifestyles. It is not unusual to see one twin looking older and sicker. One is aging faster because of factors affecting the epigenome, damaging the genes and DNA. These observations raise the question that it is not just our DNA that drives how or why we age. What happens to the driver or epigenome determines our health and lifespan.

My book will help you modify your diet and lifestyle to positively influence the factors and forces that impact your epigenome, which, as we have said before, is responsible for what happens to your genes and DNA. My basic DRESS-SS prescription is your baseline to get what Tithonus, the Greek myth character, could not: a long life with lasting health. As science advances, more factors and interventions will allow us to enjoy a life free of chronic diseases prevalent as we age. We already have what Tithonus didn't have—more knowledge about our diets and epigenome. Methionine and BCAA restriction are two ways to start this life extension and health process immediately. People who adopt diets restricting the above amino acids and a wellness lifestyle shouldn't dread reaching old age or living longer. Remember, Tithonus didn't know these factors, but you do now.

Is Aging a Disease?

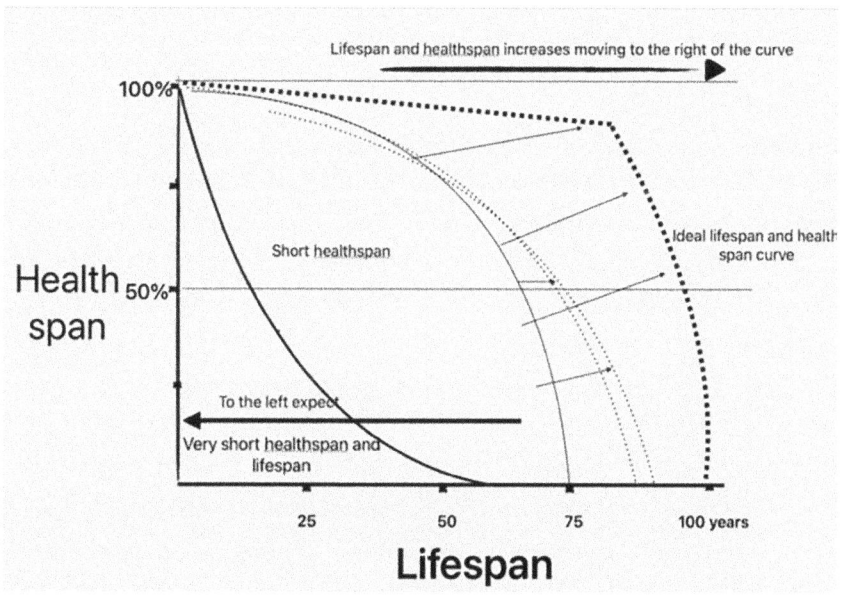

Graphic 1

Most scientists today believe that aging is, in fact, a disease. Even if you exercise, eat well, and care for yourself, you may notice changes in your body that seem difficult to control. All these changes are symptoms and signs of aging, as with any disease. Organs and systemic functions appear to decline about 1% per year, depending upon your lifestyle. Some people age faster than others, particularly if they have inadequate diets, unhealthy behavior, or a disruptive lifestyle. If someone is exposed to toxic substances, smokes, drinks alcohol regularly, abuses narcotics, has poor sleeping habits, and has constant and detrimental stress, they will age biologically faster. They may even look older than their biological age. Look around-if you see people of the same chronological age and you look older, it is most likely you are experiencing the expression of harmful genes, developing more mutations exposing you to early cancers, loss of your cognitive function, and overall decline of most of your physiological processes. Typically, all humans suffer some degree of loss of function.

In Graphic 1, I explain health span and lifespan. Far to the right of the graphic, the ideal curve shows that an optimal health span is possible until the end of the lifespan. For this to happen, anyone programmed to live 100 years may reach such an Age with minimal morbidity or disability. Take, for instance, muscle wasting, also known as sarcopenia. By age 80, a person may have lost 50% of the muscle mass and strength. The weakness at this age is the cause of many falls affecting older people. Such deficiency is preventable. If you exercise regularly, strengthening the muscles to maintain strength and mass, you may reach age 80 with minimal losses.

The same may happen with cognitive activities. Keeping your intellectual functions engaged by learning, becoming social, reading, writing, composing puzzles, or a stimulating mental activity will improve the neurological connections and production of neurotransmitters to improve cognitive function. Exercise and social activity also contribute to improving neurological connectivity. Exposure to bad diets, mainly those rich in sugars and carbohydrates, accelerates the production of AGEs or glycation agents, free radicals, and the development of plaques damaging the nerve cells. Amyloid plaques are typical in Alzheimer's and people with diabetes and diets rich in carbohydrates. This disease affects people in their later years and is known as Diabetes 3. Understanding the decline of hormones produced by the hypothalamus is essential since this organ is a central regulator of many biological functions that decline as the individual ages.

What Role the Hypothalamus play in the Aging Process?

Aging brings about significant changes in the **hypothalamus**, a vital brain region responsible for maintaining overall **homeostasis** in the body. Let's break down how aging impacts this crucial area:

1. **Sensitivity Decline**: With advanced age, the **hypothalamus** becomes less responsive to various **feedback signals**. These signals regulate temperature, hunger, thirst, and sleep. **As the sensitivity wanes, the hypothalamus may struggle to maintain balance in these essential bodily processes.**
2. **Hormonal Dysregulation**: The hypothalamus is the source and target of many hormones and factors contributing to overall homeostasis. However, aging disrupts this delicate balance. For instance:
    - The cessation of the hypothalamus-pituitary-gonadal (HPG) function triggers a cascade of effects, including loss of muscle tone, reduced bone density (related to the HP-growth hormone/IGF axis), weakened immune responses (linked to the HP-adrenal axis), circadian rhythms resulting in sleep alterations, lack of sleep, reductions in reduction of growth hormone to restore vitality and energy, decrease stress response, energy homeostasis, including food intake, fat storage, energy expenditure, body temperature regulation, and even cognitive decline.
3. **Gene Expression Changes**: Several aging-related genes identified within the hypothalamus over the years play crucial roles in nutrient sensing, metabolic regulation, energy balance, reproductive function, and stress adaptation. Examples include
4. **Mitochondrial Involvement**: Inside the mitochondria, **succinate**—a key intermediate in the Krebs cycle—

plays a significant role. Succinate oxidation within mitochondria provides potent energy output. Interestingly, extra-mitochondrial succinate activates various signaling pathways (via the **succinate receptor SUCN1 or GPR91**) in peripheral tissues, including the hypothalamus. One of its actions stabilizes cellular stress conditions by inducing the transcriptional regulator **HIF-1α. This mechanism suggests that succinate might help counteract the gradual functional decline associated with cellular senescence and systemic aging.**

In summary, the hypothalamus, which functions as a central hub for maintaining balance, undergoes intricate changes during aging. <u>Understanding these processes can shed light on age-related health challenges and potential interventions.</u> Hormonal equilibrium as we age is essential. Many women and men neglect to check their hormone levels when they begin to decline, for women with the onset of menopause and men with a decline of testosterone or andropause. The untreated decline of hormones contributes to premature aging of the skin and the production of toxic senescent substances by dying cells that, when released, affect all other organs.

Is Skin Aging an Early Sign of Premature Aging and Health Decline?

Skin aging is a disease. The same is valid for aging. Medicine has been behind, calling aging a disease. Osteoporosis is a disease now, but it wasn't until 1994 that studies showed that taking Vitamin D and Calcium combined with exercise this condition was preventable. Before 1994, osteoporosis was considered a normal process of aging. We now know that doctors can treat osteoporosis, leading to many fractures in older people, and it is not necessarily part of aging because they are preventable. Premature wrinkles and skin aging are now going through the same process. We are learning that many environmental factors, as well as internal factors, contribute to aging skin. Recent research shows that as the skin ages, it releases toxic chemicals that affect all the organs around the body, leading to premature aging. Wrinkles may not be the result of aging but the driver of it. The skin is the largest organ of our bodies and it serves as a barrier between our inner world and the outside. The skin has many other functions, too. It has a role in immunity and the production of Vitamin D, which is involved in multiple vital chemical reactions in our organs.

The skin interacts with our hypothalamus in regulating our temperature, hydration, water balance, healing of wounds as part of the inflammatory response to injury or infection, and production of melanin, a pigment to protect the skin. The skin consists of two main layers: the epidermis and the dermis. The epidermis is our first line of defense against the outside world. Its surface is a layer of dead cells forming a rugged, waterproof, very flexible shell, which is replaced continuously by a layer of stem cells below. This layer is rich in hyaluronic acid that helps destroy harmful free radicals from the cell metabolism and hydrate the epidermis. The dermis consists of connective tissue that contains proteins like collagen and elastin to provide structural support and more elasticity and strength. This layer also contains fibroblasts, which produce collagen, elastin, and hyaluronic acid, essential in wound healing.

As skin ages, it degenerates. In the epidermis, stem cell activity slows down, and more cells enter a zombie-like state called senescence. The immune system typically removes these old cells when young or healthy. Still, as we age or the skin is under a great deal of stress, these cells produce a cocktail of inflammatory cytokines and other toxic chemicals that are transported to the entire body, causing damage to other organs and tissues. When the fibroblasts in the dermis decline, collagen and elastin production decline, too. All these changes in the epidermis and dermis contribute to further wrinkling and sagging. The scaffolds of collagen and elastin crumble, producing wrinkles and damaging the skin's integrity.

The aging process worsens due to external forces such as pollution, smoking, poor diets, and UV light. Exposure to UV light accelerates skin aging unless the skin is protected. There are two kinds of UV radiation. UVA penetrates the epidermis and the dermis. UVB radiation only goes as deep as the epidermis. Both types of UV radiation cause damage to collagen and elastin, which becomes degraded and fragmented. This type of radiation is called photoaging. UV also damages the DNA of skin cells, leading to skin cancers and progressive production of senescent cells. Evidence shows skin age correlates with general health, longevity, and risk of illnesses and death. A study from Unilever and several universities found that facial photoaging correlates with the risk of cardiovascular disease in people in their 60s. Another study in 2015 of people in their 70s correlated with the likelihood of dying over the next 12 years using photographs taken years earlier. Another recent study found that people who look facially younger than their actual age were less likely to have cataracts, osteoporosis, age-related hearing loss, COPD, and better cognitive function. Young skin is a sign of being biologically younger even though a person is chronologically older.

When I wrote my first book, my wife's youthful appearance served as my significant inspiration. Her skin looks young, which makes her look twenty to thirty years younger than her chronological age. Her diet is low in carbohydrates and rich in antioxidants and anti-inflammatory foods. In addition, she takes care of her skin against the elements with sunblock, hyaluronic acid applied twice a day, and moisturizers. She drinks at least six glasses of water daily for better hydration. Her regimen also includes supplements like Turmeric, Boswellia, and DHEA to control chronic inflammation. She maintains her hormones in equilibrium, including thyroid, estrogen, and testosterone. She also doesn't drink alcohol or smoke. All these factors are signs of healthy skin and low production of toxic inflammatory cytokines from senescent cells. I believe that reversing skin aging also reverses whole-body aging and provides a guide for a healthier lifestyle and longevity.

Eczema, frequent skin rashes, and dark spots are signs of a chronic inflammatory response. Food sensitivities and a leaky gut usually contribute to an autonomic disease responsible for these complaints.

Understanding the physiology of cutaneous itching sheds light on the multifactorial altered functionality of aged skin. Xerosis and associated pruritis are the most commonly reported skin complaints of the elderly population. Chronic idiopathic pruritus most commonly occurs in older individuals, and this condition shares common molecular alterations with inflammatory atopic dermatitis. In the skin of affected patients, type 2 cytokines can directly activate sensory neurons, and chronic itch is associated with neuronal IL-4 receptor alpha and Janus kinase (JAK)-1 signaling.

The toxic effects of aging skin and a leaky gut compound the challenges faced by many people as they age. Add to this state of chronic inflammation environmental factors, alcohol intake, smoking, drug use, insomnia, stress, poor diets rich in carbs, saturated animal fats, and deficient nutrients; an individual under these circumstances is aging at a fast rate. No wonder why when a virus like COVID-19 infects this person, they feel worse and may die prematurely from this illness. These individuals are victims of the perfect "cytokine storm," where their system is overwhelmed by the toxic effects of an excessive number of inflammatory cytokines.

I warn those who spend lots of time outdoors exercising or working day after day exposed to sunlight. Skin not protected with sunblock, over 30 SPF produces extensive cytokines. The longer your skin receives UV radiation, the more significant the damage to the stem cells in your epidermis and fibroblasts. Remember that excessive exercise generates large numbers of free radicals, which contribute to causing damage to your cell's DNA, generating mutations and the possibility of cancers. Skin cancer and melanomas are common in people with prolonged exposure to UV radiation for a long time. Sunscreen products are for daily application to the body for a lifetime. Companies that produce sunscreen ingredients and products must ensure thorough testing for potential short-term and long-term health effects. This testing includes toxicity testing for irritation and skin allergies, as well as testing for skin absorption and the potential to cause cancer, disrupt the hormone system, and cause harm during reproduction and development.

In 2021, the U.S. Food and Drug Administration, which governs sunscreen safety, proposed its most recent updates to sunscreen regulations. A review found that only two ingredients, zinc oxide, and titanium dioxide, could be classified as safe and effective based on the currently available information.

Twelve other ingredients listed as not generally recognized as safe and effective due to insufficient data: avobenzone, cinoxate, dioxybenzone, ensulizole, homosalate, meradimate, octinoxate, octisalate, octocrylene, oxybenzone, padimate O, and sulisobenzone. It's advisable to avoid sunblock creams or lotions that contain these ingredients.

The FDA has required additional safety data because of health concerns, and studies by the agency show that these ingredients pass through the skin. However, in recent years, many studies have raised concerns about the endocrine-disrupting effects of three ingredients: homosalate, avobenzone, and oxybenzone.

In 2021, the European Commission also published preliminary opinions on the safety of three organic ultraviolet (UV) filters: <u>oxybenzone</u>, <u>homosalate</u>, and <u>octocrylene</u>. It found that these ingredients were unsafe and proposed limiting their concentrations to 2.2 percent for oxybenzone and 1.4 percent for homosalate.

U.S. sunscreen manufacturers are legally allowed to use these two chemicals at concentrations up to 6 and 15 percent, respectively. Hundreds of sunscreens made in the U.S. have concentrations far above the European Commission's recommendations.

According to studies published by the FDA, the ingredients oxybenzone, octinoxate, octisalate, octocrylene, homosalate, and avobenzone are all systemically absorbed into the body after just one use. The agency also detected these agents on the skin and in the blood weeks after their application.

Can a Healthier Lifestyle increase our Lifespan?

Yes. The objective of this book is to help you improve your health and achieve a longer lifespan. The curve in Graphic 1 illustrates this concept.

Many negative factors contribute to the aging process. When everything is toxic inside and outside, the epigenome may become overwhelmed and damage the mitochondria and nuclear DNA. Persistent toxicity may lead to catastrophic failure, resulting in disease, health decline, cell senescence, increased morbidity, and total collapse and death.

Graphic 1 shows how a decreased health span is closely associated with a reduced lifespan. The small arrows pointing to the right towards the ideal curve reflect actions you can take to prevent premature aging and death. My DRESS-SS prescription is a way to reverse the trend of early morbidity, disability, and early death when you follow the arrows to the right.

How can we determine our biological age?

Epigenome and genome

External and internal factors influence epigenome

Positive factors Diet, Rest, Exercise, Sleep, Stress, Sexuality, Spirituality (DRESS-SS)

Negative factors Toxic environmental factors, chemical, chronic inflammation, mutations, unhealthy behaviors, bad diets and unhealthy lifestyles

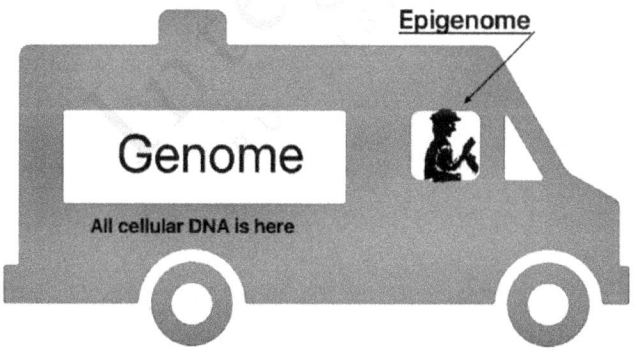

At the cellular level, the epigenome activates proteins to turn genes off and on

Epigenome is the driver involved in DNA methylation to determine the expression of genes

Graphic 2

Your birthday reflects your chronological age but not your biological age. Today, it is possible to determine the age of your biological clock. Scientists can test specific markers in a lab to determine your biological age. Also, today, it is possible to assess the length of your telomeres, which are the end caps of your chromosomes that shorten as you age. Steve Horvath, a scientist at the University of California, developed an epigenetic clock based on your biological age. There are other biological clocks. One important clock for assessing our biological clock is the methylation clock. A biological clock can determine our age and track improvements through a careful program to reverse aging.

Graphic 2 shows that the epigenome is the driver of the genome. By removing chemical tags or bookmarks, proteins above the genes can turn the genes on or off.

Genes can express themselves (turned on) or silenced (turned off) by adding or removing a methyl tag. Positive and negative factors affect the epigenome, affecting the proteins above the genes to perform specific activities.

The epigenome is the key to understanding how to unlock or influence the secrets of healthy aging, morbidity, and longevity. The genome is like the hardware, and the epigenome is like the software.

At the cellular level, epigenetics is the activity of a group of proteins constantly communicating with the DNA. Methyl groups made up of carbon and three hydrogen atoms are the tags connecting the strands of DNA. The proteins of the epigenome work as an analog code to tell the DNA to make proteins. The strands of DNA use amino acids to create sequences identified by letter (CTAG). These sequences form two strands that twist around and wrap around spools called Histones, forming clusters of eight called Nucleosomes. When a methyl tag attaches to the DNA strands mediated by an enzyme, the process is called methylation. Methylation is a chemical reaction that happens constantly and is one of the most critical reactions inside the cells.

Methylation allows the formation of:

- Neurotransmitters Production of white and red cells Hormone metabolism Production of energy in all cells, but especially muscles Activation of precursors in many chemical reactions Production of DNA DNA repair DNA expression Equilibrium and health of the entire cellular system

Methylation slows down as we get older, but this is reversible. One way to determine abnormal methylation is to assess homocysteine levels in blood. Elevations of homocysteine are indications that the methylation process is impaired and, most of the time, is associated with high cardiovascular risks of heart disease, neurological problems, anxiety, or depression. As we can see, DNA methylation plays a vital role in epigenetic expression. DNA methylation is a powerful influencer of cell division, besides other chemical tags involved in chemical reactions at the DNA level. Decreased DNA methylation plays an essential role in developing chronic diseases and aging.

Graphic 2 represents a truck loaded with all the DNA inside the cell. Like hardware can't be modified or changed without the influence of the driver, the epigenome. DNA can change through editing only under special procedures like CRISPR editing. Removing sequences of amino acids in the chromosomes can cure diseases or revert mutations.

Can we stop or prevent a family disease from developing as we age?

As we can see, biological aging and disease are consequences of errors in coding. It appears the epigenome is under constant negative and positive factors. At some point, these influences may allow abnormal genes to express the illness running in some families. Take diabetes as an example—families with a gene predisposing to type 2 develop diabetes. Years or decades later, they become sick depending on the high sugars in the diet. However, if a person in this lineage of families decides to decrease and substantially limit the consumption of sugars and carbohydrates, they can prevent the expression of this gene. In other words, the epigenome will turn off the defective gene, and diabetes will not develop.

My wife has been an example and inspiration in this matter. Her family, on both sides, has a strong history of diabetes. Grandparents, parents, siblings, cousins, and even our son have diabetes. She is the only one in the family who has no diabetes. Early in our marriage, we committed to restricting the consumption of sugars or foods rich in carbohydrates. This practice over several decades has worked. However, she remains vigilant. Any excess may result in an increase in her A1c or fasting blood sugar. So far, her data shows all these values under control. Such vigilance is difficult if a person lacks discipline or forgets why such a low-carb diet is necessary. This lack of understanding and discipline turns people with defective genes into people with diabetes requiring medications and, in extreme cases, insulin. Diabetes is a destructive disease. Excess sugars lead to a high production of free radicals, which triggers chronic inflammation. The elevated sugar in the blood triggers the production of insulin. Eventually, the cells develop insulin resistance. High blood sugar and insulin levels aggravate the problems. The excess sugar converts into fats, causing weight gain and metabolic syndrome. Inflammation of the blood vessels leads to cardiovascular diseases, plaque formation, and obstruction of the coronaries and cerebral blood vessels. I wonder why, decades later, such a person develops heart attacks or strokes. We have already discussed how Alzheimer's is also a consequence of such a disorder.

As I said before, my wife is an example that diabetes Type 2 is preventable in families with a strong history of diabetes. Modifying your diet can prevent the expression of defective genes responsible for chronic illness, morbidity, and short lifespans.

Examples of negative influences in your epigenome include poor and unhealthy diets rich in saturated fats and sugars, lack of exercise, insomnia or sleep deprivation, excessive stress, hormonal imbalance, harmful behaviors, exposure to toxins, and toxic environments.

Positive influences include healthy diets, fruits, and vegetables rich in polyphenols, antioxidants, and proteins. Healthy smoothies or drinks, no alcohol, frequent and vigorous exercise with moderation at least three times a week, good deep sound sleep from 7-8 hours a day, rest periods to meditate or to enjoy a short break, minimal stress and an environment free of damaging stress, and a balanced hormone system.

It would help if you did something to influence the epigenome to stop the disruptive gene from expressing. It would be best if you had a guide to help you how to confront this situation. In our first book, we offer a guide and a prescription using the word DRESS-SS as a code, which is easier to remember. Our book *"Living Longer and Reversing Aging"* explains that diet, Rest, Exercise, Sleep, Stress Management, Sexuality, and Spirituality are the keys to a healthier and longer life. This new book emphasizes eating right as the basis of a healthier life and longevity. Our book is a guide, and my DRESS-SS code is your prescription. In my code, you can turn on or turn off disruptive genes or activate good genes, extend the length of your telomeres, and enjoy a healthier life and longer lifespan.

Dr. Elizabeth Blackburn, winner of the Nobel Prize, demonstrated that it is possible to shorten or enlarge your telomeres with diets and changes in behavior.

Behavioral changes are essential to extend our lifespan. Our books are guides to help you to accomplish your goals.

A fundamental concept is to realize that foods are chemicals. They contain proteins, fats, sugars, minerals, vitamins, antioxidants, and many other chemical structures that can activate or inhibit enzymes, start chemical reactions, direct the production of proteins, hormones, new tissues, and the creation of new organs from stem cells. Cells behave like tiny chemical labs or factories that maintain and produce energy and repair the development of new tissues, proteins, and structures after severe injury or damage. This book explains how diet interacts with our digestive system, skin, hormones, and entire body for survival, health span, and longevity.

Most diseases are preventable.

Can aging-related diseases be prevented?

Certainly! **Aging-related diseases** are a significant concern as we grow older. Most diseases affecting people as they age are preventable. You could prevent lung cancer and COPD if you don't smoke. A plant-based diet, rich in antioxidants and anti-inflammatory foods, can reverse plaque and prevent the development of heart disease, coronary artery disease, and strokes. Muscle weakness, sarcopenia, and generalized weakness can be prevented by regular exercise and building muscle mass. Osteopenia and osteoporosis are preventable with vitamin D and calcium intake and exercise. Frequent breast exams, mammograms, and ultrasounds can prevent breast cancer. Prostate cancer, as well as many other cancers, have been associated with the consumption of dairy products; eliminating meat and overcooked meat precludes the development of colon cancer. Vaccination against many viruses and pneumonia prevents the growth of severe infections and pneumonia. Avoiding many processed foods and toxic additives in our foods prevents the growth of autonomic diseases, morbidity, and premature death. While complete prevention may not always be possible, some strategies and interventions can help promote healthy aging and reduce the risk of morbidity, poor health, chronic inflammation, and age-related diseases. To reach this goal, we should be ready to accept and adopt changes and the following strategies:

Healthy Lifestyle Choices:

- **Physical Activity**: Regular exercise helps maintain bodily function, cardiovascular health, and mental well-being.
- **Balanced Diet**: Eating nutrient-rich foods supports overall health and may improve brain function.
- **Avoid Smoking**: Quitting smoking reduces the risk of various diseases.
- **Moderate Alcohol Intake**: Limiting alcohol consumption promotes better health.

- **Maintain a Healthy Microbiome**: Ingesting good probiotics that enhance the protection of the intestinal wall and the production of good chemicals, hormones, peptides, and nutrients by the microbiome.

Screenings and Immunizations:

- **Regular health check-ups and Screenings**: These can detect chronic conditions early.
- **Immunizations**: Vaccines such as flu and pneumonia protect against infectious diseases.

Behavioral Interventions

- **Adherence to Healthy Behaviors**: As we age, we should adopt and maintain healthy habits and keep the brain active and engaged to prevent mental decline.
- **Early Detection**: Improved approaches for identifying age-related conditions early.

Clinical Treatments and Therapies:

- **Stem Cell Therapy**: Investigating stem cells for tissue regeneration and repair, including rejuvenation therapy.
- **Antioxidative and Anti-Inflammatory Treatments**: Eating antioxidants to prevent chronic inflammation and cellular damage with fruits and vegetables rich in antioxidants.
- **Hormone Replacement Therapy**: As we reach hormonal decline, we should treat hormonal imbalances early to maintain hormonal equilibrium and homeostasis.
- **Depletion of Senescent Cells**: As we age, cells may become a source of toxic cytokines; senolytics and supplements may be used to remove zombie cells associated with chronic inflammation.

- **Nutritional Interventions**: Eating right and exploring dietary modification supplements to compensate for dietary deficiencies and promote better health.
- **Microbiota Transplantation**: Studying gut microbiome effects, probiotics, and prebiotic supplementation.

Environmental Optimization:

- **Wearable Technologies**: Real-time monitoring of health indicators.
- **Remote Sensors and AI**: Facilitating care for older adults, including those with dementia.
- **Clean environments**: Homes free of mycotoxins and dangerous chemicals in the food chain.

We can't completely prevent aging-related diseases. Ideally, it is possible with a plan in mind. My prescription, DRESS-SS, is a way to institute interventions to guide you to significantly improve health, promote longevity, and enhance the quality of life as you age. I encourage you to read my first book, "Living Longer and Reversing Aging," for more information. This current book is an expansion of the first letter of this prescription. I will be addressing the other letters of my prescription in future books. My book about taming the fire of chronic inflammation will be available soon. Stay in touch.

CHAPTER 6

Appendix A: Healthy Smoothies and Recipes

We recommend healthy dishes made from fresh, whole plants. Avoid processed or ultra-processed foods, as they are responsible for many illnesses, premature death, and shortened longevity.

Green Delight Drink for the Family

Ingredients
- -1/2 cup kale
- -1/2 cup spinach-1/2 cup slid apples
- -1/2 banana
- -1/2 cup pineapple chunks
- -2 cups of water

Directions:

Mix all ingredients in a blender on high for one minute. Add more water to thin. This basic smoothie will help you be creative. As explained below, you can add more fruits or vegetables.

- Buy a juicer to prepare your juices from fruits and vegetables to prepare juices and soups. You can buy a blend of vegetable juice ready to use from Naked Juice Co. in any supermarket.

- Substitute bananas for 1 cup of frozen strawberries or blueberries to enjoy different flavors.
- These smoothies are a way to add vegetables to children's diets. Schools should provide these smoothies instead of sodas or juices rich in sugars since they provide a healthier blend of vegetables and fruits, which are refreshing and palatable.
- This smoothie has fiber to lower the absorption of the carbs in the fruits. Kale and spinach are rich in protein, calcium, and vitamin K, with high nutritional value. See Tables 1 and 2. Prepare this basic veggie-fruit smoothie for all your meals.

Tips for Enhancement:

- Add almond milk to make high-protein shakes to this basic smoothie.
- Add plant protein powder, liquid omega-3, and beetroot powder to increase protein, good fatty acids, and nitric oxide (NO) content. These shakes have enough protein, good fatty acids, complex carbs, fiber, minerals, and vitamins.
- Adding blueberries that have a higher content of antioxidants, this shake helps to fight free radicals.

These smoothies are anti-inflammatory and an excellent way to fight chronic inflammation. You can substitute a meal with this shake for children, active young adults, muscle builders, patients recovering from illness, surgery, or injuries, and people suffering from inflammation. Use protein from plants and avoid dairy or soy.

I also recommend brewer's yeast, available as flakes, since the flakes provide all essential amino acids and minerals like chromium, which help to improve insulin sensitivity, increase HDL, and lower triglycerides. Chromium also helps to improve acne, which is very common in adolescents.

You can enjoy these shakes more than one time a day. If you are trying to lose weight, this is a way to control your food intake. Keep carbs below 15 grams per serving if you want to lose weight. Always be aware of the glycemic index of many fruits.

Use your blender or juicer to make vegetable soups. Add favorite spices and condiments, thenheat before serving.

Drinks and Low-carb Smoothies

Morning Essentials

Ingredients
-1/2 cup fresh squeezed orange juice-One teaspoon of omega-3 fish oil or flaxseed oil (Barlean brand) that comes in different flavors. It contains 660 mg of EPA,420 mg of DHA, and 270 mg of other omega-3 fatty acids.

Directions
Mix in a glass to start your day with the essentials.

- This is a great drink to stay healthy, keep your body strong, reduce inflammation, help your body repair cell membranes and cartilage, and maintain a healthy heart. I recommend 50 percent reduced sugar orange juice, squeezed oranges, lemon juice, or diet apple juice. Fish oil and flaxseed oil are available in different flavors packed with omega-3. We prefer the Barlean brand because it offers many flavors, not fish flavor, and reduced calories.
- Vitamin C and omega-3 are two essential vital nutrients. My wife and I drink this smoothie every morning. You can add yeast flakes to add more amino acids and minerals like chromium, magnesium, calcium, and selenium. You find the Barlean brand in vitamin and health food stores.

Libido Power Smoothie

Ingredients
-1/2 watermelon -One tablespoon of shelled sunflower seeds -One teaspoon L-arginine powder -1/2 cup ice -2 cups water -One teaspoon of L-Thyrosine-1/2 squeezed lemon.

Directions

Blend at high speed for one minute.

- Watermelon is rich in citrulline and L-arginine. Both amino acids help to raise nitric oxide, a vasodilator, which in turn improves libido, lowers blood pressure, and improves circulation.
- L-thyroxine is a precursor of dopamine that helps reduce anxiety and depression.

Citrus Strawberry Smoothie

Ingredients

-1 cup squeezed orange juice-1 cup frozen strawberries-1/3 cup shelled sunflower seeds-One teaspoon of liquid omega-3 or flaxseed oil (available in many flavors)-One cup of sugar-free yogurt-1 cup water

Directions

Mix the ingredients in a blender and blend for 45 seconds at high speed. Garnish with a strawberry if desired. Add Stevia to your taste if desired.

This preparation yields 4 cups. Using more water and more sesame seeds for fiber helps to lower the carbs intake.

This smoothie is rich in vitamins A, B, B6, and E; magnesium, manganese, selenium, zinc, and copper; and omega-3 and cysteine. Plus, it has lots of antioxidants. It's great to strengthen your immune system.

Mango Sensational Smoothie

Ingredients:

-One cup of mango pulp-2 cups water-Two tablespoons sesame seeds 1 cup sugar-free yogurt-One tablespoon stevia-1 cup ice

Directions:

Mix ingredients in the blender and blend for 45 seconds at high speed.

- Sesame seeds provide fiber to decrease the carbs in a mango.
- You can buy fresh mangos or buy the pulp ready for use.

Goya Foods in the Mexican section offers many frozen fruits for juices ready to blend. Many supermarkets provide fruits and veggies already in a packet and prepared to blend. You can make your own in a plastic bag.

Try a different smoothie for each day of the week.

Mixing fruits and vegetables can provide fiber and low-carb as elements of a low-carb diet. As a rule, my wife and I are primarily vegetarians. Besides smoothies, we add fish, poultry, and eggs to our diets for a more balanced diet. Fiber is essential to lower the carb's load. I recommend you check Tables 1 and 2 for many fruits' antioxidants and carb content. If you are on a diet, keep carbs below 15 g when making smoothies. Your daily carbs should not exceed 30 g if you want to keep your weight down.

On the contrary, if you are recovering from an illness or need to gain weight, you can be more liberal with your carbs unless you have diabetes. Add plant-based powder to the smoothies for more protein to gain weight or muscle mass. I recommend plant protein rather than whey or milk protein products since they contain most of the amino acids and minerals required in a well-balanced diet and are free of antibiotics and hormones. I also recommend brewer's yeast in the form of yeast flakes or powder made from Saccharomyces cerevisiae for more amino acids and minerals like chromium and selenium. My wife and I prefer the yeast flakes from KAL found in vitamin and health food stores.

Healthy avocado, salmon toast

Ingredients:

-1/2 avocado -One slice of whole multigrain or rye bread -3-4 spinach or lettuce leaves -2-inch square of smoked salmon -One tablespoon of hummus

Toast the bread in a skillet with avocado oil.

Spread the hummus on the toast, place the veggies on top of the hummus, apply the salmon square on top, and finally apply the avocado in small slices.

This toast is rich in good fatty acids, provides protein from salmon, avocado, and hummus, and has polyphenols and antioxidants from the veggies. It's an excellent way to start your breakfast with a smoothie or a matcha latte with almond milk. If you follow our intermittent fasting recommendation, you will combine breakfast and lunch.

Healthy Desserts

Coconut Blueberry Yogurt Ingredients

Ingredients:
  -1/2 cup of Chobani Greek yogurt
  -1/2 cup of fresh blueberries

A delightful dessert is easy to prepare. Use 1/2 a cup of coconut nonfat Chobani Greek yogurt and a half cup of fresh blueberries. You can add Stevia for a sweet flavor.

This dessert is rich in antioxidants and probiotics. To add fiber, add a tablespoon of yeast flakes or powder.

Walnuts and Blueberry Cottage Cheese

Ingredients:
  -1/2 cup of low-fat cottage cheese
  -1/2 cup of walnuts
  -1/2 cup of fresh blueberries

Add half a cup of low-fat cottage cheese to half a cup of walnuts and half a cup of blueberries. This dessert is rich in antioxidants, calcium, minerals, and proteins. Add Stevia for a sweet flavor and yeast flakes for more protein.

Super Omega-3 Tofu Dessert

Ingredients:
-1-inch-thick slice of hard tofu
-One tablespoon of flax-chia blend
-One teaspoon of Stevia

Cut a thick slice of hard tofu into small squares, sprinkle with a tablespoon of the flax-chia blend from Garden of Life, add a teaspoon of Stevia and mix.

The flax-chia blend contains 5 g of fiber, omega-3, antioxidants, calcium, iron, magnesium, and other healthy minerals in vitamin and health food stores.

Brewer's Yeast Flakes Yogurt

Ingredients:
-1/2 cup of light carb-free yogurt
-One tablespoon of yeast flakes

Serve a half cup of flavored or nonflavored low-fat yogurt that contains probiotics, and add a tablespoon of yeast flakes from KAL. Add Stevia powder for additional sweetness and mix.

KAL makes Brewer's yeast flakes from Saccharomyces cerevisiae, which are rich in essential amino acids, B vitamins, minerals, and fiber.

You can find this brand of yeast flakes in vitamin and supplement stores.

Coconut-Chia Delight

Ingredients
-1 cup of almond milk
-1/2 cup chia seeds
-One teaspoon of Stevia and one teaspoon of vanilla extract

- Mix the ingredients in a jar, cover tightly, and shake the mix.
- Place the jar in the refrigerator for at least 30 minutes or leave overnight for 12 hours.
- Serve with blueberries or fruit and more Stevia for sweetness (optional).

Coconut-Chia Delight is incredible for breakfast as well.

A Healthy Salad

Nice Sleep Salad

In the evening, you can prepare a healthy salad with spinach, kale, avocado, tomatoes, almonds, walnuts, pineapple, and orange chunks. Add balsamic vinaigrette and olive oil. For more protein, add salmon or chicken. Sprinkle with Turmeric powder.

This salad contains sufficient magnesium, calcium, and L-Tryptophan, the primary amino acid and precursor of serotonin and melatonin. It helps to increase melatonin levels during the night and restore your normal circadian rhythm at night. If you want to fall asleep soon and enjoy more relaxation:

1. Add Ashwagandha powder to your salad. You can drink Chamomile with Lavender tea or an anti-stress tea with Ashwagandha.
2. Avoid caffeine and alcohol if you have insomnia or difficulty sleeping.
3. Avoid refined sugars and too many carbs at night since they raise insulin levels, interfering with sleep.
4. Avocado is an excellent fruit, but unlike many fruits, it doesn't contain sugars. It contains good fatty acids, proteins, vitaminš A, B, C, E, and K, calcium, monounsaturated fats (MUFA), magnesium, potassium, fiber, zinc, iron, folate, and antioxidants. Avocado contains three times as much fiber as Asparagus, Apples, and Melons. Avocados decrease your cravings for food since they take longer to digest. When combined with lemon juice and egg whites,

you can make a paste for a facial mask to reduce wrinkles and improve skin elasticity. Because of the fiber and healthy fatty acids, avocados slow down the absorption of carbohydrates, stabilizing blood sugar in people with diabetes.

Appendix B: Resources

Screening and Blood Testing:

Quest and Lab Corp are national laboratories most doctors use for almost any kind of lab testing.

1. Quest Diagnostics
   Quest offers comprehensive lab services and testing across various health areas.
   Website: www.questdiagnostics.com
2. Lab Corp
   A national laboratory offering extensive lab testing, commonly used by doctors.
   Website: www.labcorp.com
3. Life Extension
   This company offers a variety of tests without needing a prescription on a cash basis through Lab Corp.
   Website: www.lifeextension.com
4. Private MD Labs
   Provides lab testing services directly to consumers without a doctor's prescription.
   Website: www.privatemdlabs.com

APPENDIX B: RESOURCES

Telomere Testing:

1. Telomere diagnostic
   Provides telomere length testing to assess cellular aging.
   Website: www.teloyears.com

DNA testing:

1. Ancestry
   Offers DNA testing services for discovering family heritage and genetic makeup.
   Website: ancestry.com
2. 23andMe
   Provides genetic testing services for health, ancestry, and wellness insights.
   Website: www.23andme.com

Genetic testing1. Mayo Clinic
   Provides extensive genetic testing and medical services for a wide range of conditions.
   Website: www.mayoclinic.org

Epigenetic and Biological Clock Testing:

1. Epimorphy
   Offers DNA methylation testing to evaluate biological age.
   Website: www.myDNAage.com2. TrueAge Epigenetic Test Kit
   Provides epigenetic testing to assess biological aging based on DNA methylation.
   Website: www.trudiagnostic.com

BIBLIOGRAPHY AND SELECTED REFERENCES

American Diabetes Association. n.d. "Glycemic Index and Diabetes." www.diabetes.org/food-and-fitness/food/what-can-i-eat/understanding-carbohydrates/glycemic-index-and-diabetes.html?loc=ff-slabnav. Accessed May 18, 2016.

Bodkin, Henry. 2018 "Atkins Diet May Cause Heart Failure." *The Telegraph*, May 29, 2018. https://www.telegraph.co.uk/science/2018/05/29/atkins-diet-may-cause-heart-failure-major-new-protein-study/.

Bergouignan, Audrey. 2016. "Effect of Frequent Interruptions of Prolonged Sitting on Self-Perceived Levels of Energy, Mood, Food Cravings and Cognitive Function." *International Journal of Behavioral Nutrition and Physical Activity,* Nov. 3, 2016. www.ijbnpa.biomedcentral.com/articles/10.1186/s12966-016-0437-z.

Blackburn, Elizabeth, PhD, and Elissa Epel, PhD. 2016. *The Telomere Effect.* New York: Grand Central Publishing.

Braverman, Eric R., MD. 2011. *Younger Brain, Sharper Mind.* New York: Rodale, Inc.

Brody, Jane E. 2016. "The Fight Against Obesity Begins Early." *New York Times*, July 5, 2016, D5.

Chopra Deepak, MD, and David Simon. 2001. *Grow Younger, Live Longer.* New York: Three Rivers Press.

Crowley, Chris, and H. Lodge, MD. 2007. *Younger Next Year.* New York: Workman Publishing.

Downey, Andrea. 2017. "Eating Curry Is Good for You!" www.thesun.co.uk/living/4092612/eating-curry-is-good-for-you-turmeric-helped-cancer-patient-57-beat-myeloma-after-five-years-of-treatment/. *The Sun.* Accessed July 25, 2017.

Dye, Lee. 2012. "Living Longer: Increasing Lifespan May Be in Our Control." ABC News, August 29, 2012. www.abcnews.go.com/Technology/humans-live-forever-longevity-research-suggests-longer-life/story?id=17100148.

Esmonde-White, Miranda. 2014. *Aging Backwards.* New York: Harper Collins.

Esselstyn, Caldwell B., Jr., MD. 2008. *Prevent and Reverse Heart Disease.* New York: Penguin Group, 64–71.

Genome.gov https://www.genome.gov/19016938/faq-about-genetics-disease-prevention-and-treatment/

Gibson, D., B. Cullen, R. Legerstee, K. G. Harding, and G. Schultz. 2009. "MMPs Made Easy." *Wounds International* 1, no. 1. Available from http://www.woundsinternational.com.

American Diabetes Association. n.d. "Glycemic Index and Diabetes." www.diabetes.org/food-and-fitness/food/what-can-i-eat/understanding-carbohydrates/glycemic-index-and-diabetes.html?loc=ff-slabnav. Accessed May 18, 2016.

Guay, André, and Susan Davis. 2002. "Testosterone Insufficiency Fact or Fiction?" *World Journal of Urology.* http://www.bumc.bu.edu/sexualmedicine/publications/testosterone-insufficiency-in-women-fact-or-fiction/.

Guerrero, G. P., M. M. Zago, N. O. Sawada, and M. H. Pinto. 2011. "Relationship between Spirituality and Cancer: Patient's Perspective." *Rev Bras Enferm* 64, no. 1: 53–59.

Gundry, Steven R., MD. 2017. *The Plant Paradox*. HarperCollins Publishers. New York, N.Y. Fox News. 2017. "No Fruit Juice for Kids under 1, Doctors Say." Fox News Health, May 22, 2017. www.foxnews.com/health/2017/05/22/no-fruit-juice-for-kids-under-1-doctors-say.html.

Haden, S. T., J. Glowacki, S. Hurwitz, C. Rosen, and M. S.LeBoff. 2000. "Effects of Age on Serum Dehydroepiandrosterone Sulfate, IGF-I, and IL-6 levels in Women." *Calcif Tissue Int* 66, no. 6 (June): 414–18.

Head, K. A. 1998. "Estriol: Safety and Efficacy." *Altern Med Rev*3, no. 2 (April): 101–13.

Heid Markham, O'Connor Siobhan, Editor. Secrets of living longer. 21-25. 2015 Time Inc. Books

Horner, Christine, MD. 2016. *Radiant Health Ageless Beauty*. San Diego: Elgea Publishing.

Hotze Steve, MD. *Hormones, Health, and Happiness*. 2013. Published by Advantage Media Group. Charleston, S.C.

Hyman, Mark, M.D. 2016. *Eat Fat, Get Thin*. New York: Little Brown and Company.

Jenkins, J. A. 2016. *Disrupt Aging*. First Edition. New York: Public Affairs.

Ironson, G., G. F. Solomon, E. G. Balbin, et al. 2002. The Ironson-Woods Spirituality/Religiousness Index Is Associated with Long Survival, Health Behaviors, Less Distress, and Low Cortisol in People with HIV/AIDS." *Ann Behav Med* 24, no. 1:34–48.

Kalamian Miriam, EdM, MS, CNS.2017. *Keto for Cancer.* Chelsea Green Publishing.

Kolata, Gina. 2016. "Diabetes and Your Diet: The Low-Carb Debate." *New York Times*, September 16, 2016. www.nytimes.com/2016/09/16/health/type-2-diabetes-low-carb-diet.html Accessed September 9, 2016.

Kramer, Leslie. 2017. "One-Third of Americans Are Headed for Diabetes, and They Don't Even Know It." CNBC.com, August 17, 2017. www.medicalxpress.com/news/2016-07-fruit-vegetables-substantially-happiness.html.

Kummer, Sebastian, MD, Derik Hermsen, MD, and Felix Distelmaier, MD. 2016. "Biotin Treatment Mimicking Grave's Disease." Massachusetts Medical Society, August 18, 2016. www.nejm.org/doi/full/10.1056/NEJMc1602096?query=endocrinology

Larimore, W. L., M. Parker, and M. Crowther. 2002. "Should Clinicians Incorporate Positive Spirituality into their Practices? What Does the Evidence Say?" *Ann Behav Med* 24, no. 1: 69–73.

Lawler-Row, K. A., and J. Elliott. 2009. "The Role of Religious Activity and Spirituality in the Health and Well-Being of Older Adults." *J Health Psychol* 14, no. 1: 43–52.

Longo, Valter, PhD. 2018. *The Longevity Diet.* New York: Penguin & Random House LLC, 214–16.

LowDog, Tieraona, MD. 2016. *Fortify Your Life.* Washington, DC: National Geographic Society.

Mayo Clinic. https://www.mayoclinic.org/diseases-conditions/menopause/in-depth/hormone-therapy/ART-20046372. May 24, 2018. Hormone therapy: Is it right for you?

McCall, Becky. 2017. "Vitamin D Supplements May Raise Sex Hormone Levels in Men." *Medscape*, June 01, 2017. European Congress of Endocrinology (ECE) (2017).

Mercola, Joseph. 2017. *Fat for Fuel*. Hay House Inc. Carlsbad, California.

Meyer, Joyce. 2015. *The Mind Connection*. New York: Faith Words Hachette Book Group.

Mizushima N. Autophagy: process and function. *Gen Dev.* 2007;21(22):2861-2873.

McVay, M. R. 2002. "Medicine and Spirituality: A Simple Path to Restore Compassion in Medicine." *SDJ Med* 55, no. 11: 487–91.

Morales, A. J., J. J. Nolan, J.C. Nelson, and S. S. Yen. 1994. "Effects of Replacement Dose of Dehydroepiandrosterone in Men and Women of Advancing Age." *J Clin Endocrinol Metab* 78, no. 6 (June): 1360–67.

Murphy Helen editor 10.01.2018. "Is Your Nitric Oxide Supplement Effective?" www.consumereview.org/nitric-oxide/nitric-oxide-supplement-effective/.

Murray, Michael, ND. 2017. *The Magic of Food*. New York: Atria Books, Simon &Schuster Inc.

National Institutes of Health (NIH) Office of Dietary Supplements. 2018. "Vitamin E: Fact Sheet for Health Professionals." https://ods.od.nih.gov/factsheets/VitaminE-HealthProfessional/.

Nelson, C. J., B. J. Rosenfeld, W. Breitbart, and M. Galietta. 2002. "Spirituality, Religion, and Depression in the Terminally Ill." *Psychosomatics* 43, no. 3: 213–20.

Noto H., A. Goto, T. Tsujimoto, and M. Noda. 2013. "Low-Carbohydrate Diets and All-Cause Mortality: A Systematic Review and Meta-Analysis of Observational Studies." *PLoS ONE* 8, no. 1: e55030. https://doi.org/10.1371/journal.pone.0055030.

Park Alice, O'Connor Siobhan. *How to live to be 100.* Secrets of living longer. Time Inc Books. 2015.

Reader's Digest Best Health. n.d. "40 Foods High in Antioxidants." Originally, it was called "Anti-Oxidant-Rich Fare" in *Best Health Magazine* (January/February 2009), accessed March 6, 2018. www.besthealthmag.ca/best-eats/nutrition/40-foods-high-in-antioxidants/.

Reivich, Karen, and Andrew Shatte. 2002. *The Resilience Factor.* NJ: Bright & Happy Books, LLC.

Renner, Ben. 2017. "Artificial Sweeteners Stimulate Fat Growth, Harmful to Metabolism, Study Finds." December 13, 2017. www.studyfinds.org/sweeteners-fat-growth-obesity/.

Reynolds, Gretchen. 2017. "Work. Walk 5 Minutes. Work." *New York Times*, January 3, 2017, D4. www.nytimes.com/2016/12/28/well/move/work-walk-5-minutes-work.html?_r=0.

Romanoski, Anya. 2018. "Ketogenic Diet: Which patients benefit?" *Medscape.* https://www.medscape.com/viewarticle/894041_4. Accessed March 24, 2018.

Salas-Salvadó, Jordi, et al. 2016. "Protective Effects of the Mediterranean Diet on Type 2 Diabetes and Metabolic Syndrome." *The Journal of Nutrition* 146, no. 4: 920S–927S. *PMC*. Web. March 5, 2018.

Sesink, Aloys L. A., Denise S. M. L. Termont, Jan H. Kleibeukerand Roelof Van der Meer. 1999. "Red Meat and Colon Cancer." *Cancer Research* (November). http://cancerres.aacrjournals.org/content/59/22/5704.

Sheldrick, Giles. 2016. "Eat Nuts to Live Longer." Accessed December 6, 2016. www.express.co.uk/life-style/health/739777/Eat-nuts-live-longer-doctors-prescribe-fight-killer-diseases-heart-disease-cancer-obesity.

Sleiman, Dana, Marwa R. Al-Badri, and Sami T. Azar. 2015. "Effect of Mediterranean Diet in Diabetes Control and Cardiovascular Risk Modification: A Systematic Review." *Frontiers in Public Health* 3: 69. *PMC*. Web. March 5, 2018.

"Spirituality." www.umm.edu/health/medical/altmed/treatment/spirituality. February 1, 2018.

Steingold, Daniel. 2017. "Study: Artificial Sweeteners Linked to Weight Gain, Other Health Problems." July 17, 2017. www.studyfinds.org/artificial-sweeteners-weight-gain-heart/.

Taubes, Gary. 2016. *The Case Against Sugar*. New York: Alfred A Knopf Publisher, a division of Penguin Random House, LLC., 258–262.

Tay, J., Luscombe-Marsh, ND, C. H. Thompson, M. Noakes, J. D. Buckley, G. A. Wittert, W. S. Yancy Jr., and G. D. Brinkworth, G.D. 2015 "Comparison of Low- and High-Carbohydrate Diets for Type 2 Diabetes Management: A Randomized Trial." *The American Journal of Clinical Nutrition* 102, 780–90. http://dx.doi.org/10.3945/ajcn.115.112581.

Weber, Robert, PhD, and Carol Orsborn, PhD. 2015. *The Spirituality of Age*. Rochester, VT: Park Street Press.

Young, Anthony, MD. 2016. *The Age Fix*. New York: Grand Central Life & Style.

ADDITIONAL BOOKS RESEARCHED

Attia, Peter., MD. 2023. *Outlive.* Harmony Books an imprint of Random House. NY.

Barnard, Neal D., MD. 2024. *The Power Foods Diet.* Hachette Book Group, Inc. NY.

Buettner, Dan.,2023. *The Blue Zones, Secrets for Living Longer.* National Geographic Partners, LLC. Washington DC

Cordain, Loren., *PhD. The Paleo Diet.* 2011 revised edition. Houghton Mifflin Harcourt Publishing. NY

Davis, William., MD.2022. *Super Gut.* Hachette Book Group Inc.

Fuhrman, Joel., MD. 2020. *Eat for Life.* Harper Collins Publishers, NY.

Gittleman, Ann Louise., 2021. *Radical Longevity.* Hachette Book Group.

Greger, Michael., MD. 2023. *How Not to Age.* Flatiron Books. NY. Fitzgerald, Kara., ND. 2022. *Younger You.* Hachette Books. NY.

Li, William W., MD. 2019. *Eat to Beat Disease.* Hachette Books. NY.

Lyon, Gabrielle., MD. 2023. *Forever Young.* Simon&Schuster. NY.

Oz, Mehmet., MD. 2017. *Food Can Fix It.* Simon & Schuster. NY.

Pedre, Vincent., MD. 2023. *The Gutsmart Protocol.* 2023. BenBella Books, Inc. Tx.

Reference Articles

Digestive system

https://my.clevelandclinic.org/health/body/7041-digestive-system
https://www.webmd.com/digestive-disorders/synbiotics-what-to-know
https://my.clevelandclinic.org/health/body/the-gut-brain-connection

Microbiome

https://gutfriendlybites.com/gut-microbiome/
https://www.microbiometimes.com/half-of-all-commonly-used-drugs-profoundly-affecting-the-gut-microbiome-warn-experts/
https://www.microbiometimes.com/half-of-all-commonly-used-drugs-profoundly-affecting-the-gut-microbiome-warn-experts/
https://www.microbiometimes.com/half-of-all-commonly-used-drugs-profoundly-affecting-the-gut-microbiome-warn-experts/
https://health.clevelandclinic.org/what-are-prebiotics/
https://www.webmd.com/healthy-aging/best-probiotic-strains-older-adults
https://www.dailyhealthcures.com/food-nutrition/what-are-the-best-probiotics-supplements/
https://www.dailyhealthcures.com/food-nutrition/what-are-the-best-probiotics-supplements/
https://health.clevelandclinic.org/how-to-pick-the-best-probiotic-for-you/?ref=blog.vitable.com.au
https://vitaliboost.com/quizzes/which-probiotic-is-right-for-me-quiz/
https://health.clevelandclinic.org/butyrate-benefits/

https://www.plixlife.com/blog/what-are-probiotics-pre-and-probiotic-capsules-dosage-their-uses-benefits-dosage/
https://www.supermarketguru.com/articles/wild-salmon-a-top-food-for-your-heart/

Vitamins and Supplements

https://nutritionsource.hsph.harvard.edu/vitamin-a/
https://elderberryholistichealth.com/the-importance-of-vitamin-a/
https://www.hsph.harvard.edu/nutritionsource/biotin-vitamin-b7/?ref=blog.vitable.com.au
https://scientificdiet.org/2022/09/vitamin-b9-deficiency-linked-to-higher-dementia-risk/
https://nutritionsource.hsph.harvard.edu/vitamin-b12/?ref=tomecontroldesusalud.com
https://justvegan.co.za/2022/03/02/vitamins-what-you-should-know/
http://anandabodh.com/shop/2022/02/20/vitamin-b12-deficiency-and-sources/
https://nutritionaldirect.com/why-vitamin-c-is-important-what-it-does-to-our-body/
https://wellbeing-support.com/just-ten-minutes-sunlight-day-can-help-prevent-baby-getting-asthma/
https://www.beehivestrong.com/group/beehive-strong-group/discussion/8427ffc0-7251-4c09-85f3-5f6a949a1522
https://thedrswolfson.com/best-magnesium-heart/
https://www.eisonreports.com/best-magnesium-supplement-for-kids/
https://www.brunel.net/en-au/blog/life-sciences/how-essential-minerals-are-mined-for-our-health
https://www.webmd.com/diet/health-benefits-msm
https://avesis.gazi.edu.tr/yayin/44149bf0-27ba-4902-8180-7f5b639e6d79/resveratrol-a-double-edged-sword-in-health-benefits
https://astroflav.com/blogs/home/8-supplements-that-reduce-inflammation
https://www.metsicare.com/post/10-natural-anti-inflammatory-supplements-backed-by-science

https://www.mdpi.com/2072-6643/16/5
https://www.alive.com/beauty/age-defying-antioxidants/
https://thewaytoeat.ca/2014/07/14/how-plant-based-diets-may-extend-our-lives/
https://audreylaureltonrdn.com/articles/reprogramming-your-body/
https://www.believebig.org/tag/sunscreen/
https://cancercenterforhealing.com/alternative-medicine-for-leukemia/

Additional articles researched

Comparison of cardiovascular risk factors between Sri Lankans living in Kandy and Oslo | BMC Public Health | Full Text. https://bmcpublichealth.biomedcentral.com/articles/10.1186/1471-2458-10-654

KETONES IDEAL FUEL FOR BODY | Interstellar Blends | Activate Your Super Powers! https://theinterstellarplan.com/2016/03/ketones-ideal-fuel-for-body/

Cancer and diabetes: The connection is in your DNA. https://www.cancercenter.com/community/blog/2021/05/diabetes-cancer

Top Reasons a Plant-based Diet Is Good for You - The Presence Portal. https://www.thepresenceportal.com/should-you-go-for-a-plant-based-diet/

Plant-Based Dietitian Guide. https://dietitiansuccesscenter.com/plant-based-dietitian/

How Long Does It Take For Ozempic To Work - Flatten the Curve. https://flattenthecurve.com/how-long-does-it-take-for-ozempic-to-work/

Best Oxidative Stress Panel Treatment In Dubai | German Medical Center. https://gmcdhcc.com/medical--services-treatment/oxidative-stress-panel/

Cancer and diabetes: The connection is in your DNA. https://www.cancercenter.com/community/blog/2021/05/diabetes-cancer

Tips on Controlling Inflammation to Help Improve Chronic Pain. https://themighty.com/topic/chronic-pain/control-inflammation-from-food-medication-chronic-pain/

"United States: FDA Approves Integra Omnigraft Dermal Regeneration Matrix to Treat Diabetic Foot Ulcers." MENA Report, vol., no., 2016, p. n/a.

Dairy Consumption and Cancers of the Prostate and Colon. https://nutritionfacts.org/blog/dairy-consumption-and-cancers-of-the-prostate-and-colon/

Digestive System: Function, Organs & Anatomy. https://my.clevelandclinic.org/health/body/7041-digestive-system

- Carabotti M, Scirocco A, Maselli MA, Severi C. The gut-brain axis: interactions between enteric microbiota, central and enteric nervous systems (https://www.ncbi.nlm.nih.gov/pmc/articles/PMC4367209/). Ann Gastroenterol. 2015 Apr-Jun;28(2):203-209. Corrected: Ann Gastroenterol. 2016 Apr-Jun;29(2):240. Accessed 9/20/2023.
- Dossett, Michelle. Brain-gut connection explains why integrative treatments can help relieve digestive ailments (https://www.health.harvard.edu/blog/brain-gut-connection-explains-why-integrative-treatments-can-help-relieve-digestive-ailments-2019041116411). Harvard Health Blog. Published 7/26/2023. Accessed 9/20/2023.
- Frankel, Miriam, Warren, Matt. How gut bacteria are controlling your brain (https://www.bbc.com/future/article/20230120-how-gut-bacteria-are-controlling-your-brain). BBC Future. Published 1/22/2023. Accessed 9/20/2023.
- Mayer EA, Tillisch K, Gupta A. Gut/brain axis and the microbiota (https://www.ncbi.nlm.nih.gov/pmc/articles/

- PMC4362231/). J Clin Invest. 2015 Mar 2;125(3):926-38. We accessed 9/20/2023.
- Ochoa-Repáraz J, Kasper LH. The Second Brain: Is the Gut Microbiota a Link Between Obesity and Central Nervous System Disorders? (https://www.ncbi.nlm.nih.gov/pmc/articles/PMC4798912/) CurrObes Rep. 2016 Mar;5(1):51-64. Accessed 9/20/2023.
- Psychology Today. Gut-Brain Axis (https://www.psychologytoday.com/us/basics/gut-brain-axis). Accessed 9/20/2023.
- Silburner, Joanne. Studying the link between the gut and mental health is personal for this scientist (https://www.npr.org/sections/health-shots/2023/07/08/1186092825/studying-the-link-between-the-gut-and-mental-health-is-personal-for-this-scienti). Health Shots/National Public Radio. Published 7/8/2023. Accessed 9/20/2023.

https://my.clevelandclinic.org/health/diseases/21688-food-intolerance

Journal: Biomedicines, **2018** Volume: 6 Number: 91
Resveratrol: A Double-Edged Sword in Health Benefits Authors: by **Bahare Salehi**, **Abhay Praka**Number: 91
Link: **https://www.mdpi.com/2227-9059/6/3/91**

Mensi, Martina M., et al. "Lactobacillus Plantarum PS128 and Other Probiotics in Children and Adolescents with Autism Spectrum Disorder: A Real-World Experience." Nutrients, 2021, https://doi.org/10.3390/nu13062036.

Vitamin A | The Nutrition Source | Harvard T.H. Chan School of Public Health. https://www.hsph.harvard.edu/nutritionsource/vitamin-a/

Biotin – Vitamin B7 | The Nutrition Source | Harvard T.H. Chan School of Public Health. https://www.hsph.harvard.edu/nutritionsource/biotin-vitamin-b7/

Vitamin B9 deficiency linked to higher dementia risk | Scientific Diet. https://scientificdiet.org/2022/09/vitamin-b9-deficiency-linked-to-higher-dementia-risk/

Vitamin B12, deficiency and sources - Anandabodh. http://anandabodh.com/shop/2022/02/20/vitamin-b12-deficiency-and-sources/

Why is Vitamin B12 Important? Need, Deficiency, and Sources | Lifezen. https://www.lifezen.in/article/why-is-vitamin-b12-important-need-deficiency-sources

Are Supplements Needed in a Plant-Based Diet? https://www.avancecare.com/are-supplements-needed-in-a-plant-based-diet/

Why Vitamin C Is Important & What it Does To Our Body - Nutritional Direct. https://nutritionaldirect.com/why-vitamin-c-is-important-what-it-does-to-our-body/

Buonocore, Daniela, et al. "Anti-inflammatory Dietary Interventions and Supplements to Improve Performance during Athletic Training." Journal of The American College of Nutrition, 2015, https://doi.org/10.1080/07315724.2015.1080548.

MSM: Health Benefits, Safety Information, Dosage, and More. https://www.webmd.com/diet/health-benefits-msm

Laky, Markus, et al. "Quercetin in the Prevention of Induced Periodontal Disease in Animal Models: A Systematic Review and Meta-analysis." Nutrients, 2024, https://doi.org/10.3390/nu16050735.

Ebersole, Jeffrey L., et al. "Aging, Inflammation, Immunity and Periodontal Disease." Periodontology 2000, 2016, https://doi.org/10.1111/prd.12135.

Periodontal disease as a model to study chronic inflammation in aging. - International Association for the Study of Pain (IASP).

https://www.iasp-pain.org/publications/pain-research-forum/papers-of-the-week/paper/periodontal-disease-as-a-model-to-study-chronic-inflammation-in-aging/

Matcha Tea Powder Organic. https://www.starwest-botanicals.com/product/matcha-tea-powder-organic/

Vitamin C, Vitamin D, and Zinc Could Help Fight Covid-19? https://www.connexions-tech.com/article/detail/Vitamin-C--Vitamin-D-and-Zinc-Could-Help-Fight-Covid-19-.html

Iodine | The Nutrition Source | Harvard T.H. Chan School of Public Health. https://www.hsph.harvard.edu/nutritionsource/iodine/

Selenium | The Nutrition Source | Harvard T.H. Chan School of Public Health. https://www.hsph.harvard.edu/nutritionsource/selenium/

Vitamin-B12: Introduction, Test Result, Unit, Normal Range, Test. https://medicallabnotes.com/vitamin-b12-introduction-test-result-unit-normal-range-test-method-clinical-significance-and-keynotes/

Vitamin B12, deficiency and sources - Anandabodh. http://anandabodh.com/shop/2022/02/20/vitamin-b12-deficiency-and-sources/

Eos, the Ancient Greek Goddess of the Dawn - GreekReporter.com. https://greekreporter.com/2022/12/10/eos-the-ancient-greek-goddess-of-the-dawn/

How Plant-Based Diets May Extend Our Lives – The Way To Eat. https://thewaytoeat.ca/2014/07/14/how-plant-based-diets-may-extend-our-lives/

Russell-Goldman, Eleanor, and Gëorge F. Murphy. "The Pathobiology of Skin Aging." American Journal of Pathology, 2020, https://doi.org/10.1016/j.ajpath.2020.03.007.

The Trouble with Ingredients in Sunscreens - Believe Big. https://www.believebig.org/the-trouble-with-ingredients-in-sunscreens/

5 Common Habits That Sabotage Your Self-Control | My family life. https://gsccy.com/2022/03/03/5-common-habits-that-sabotage-your-self-control/

Age-Defying Antioxidants | healthy. https://www.jinpei.net/2015/04/24/age-defying-antioxidants/

INDEX

A

acidosis 62, 73
  Diabetic ketoacidosis 62, 73
  Ketosis 62, 73
Advanced Glycation End products 35
AGEs 35, 36, 140
Aging 181
Akkermansia Municiphila 21, 43
Allergies
  foods iii, 172
  Mycotoxins 87
  testing 88
Alzheimer's disease 16, 26, 94, 106, 118, 136
Animal-based diets 20
  Bilophila bacteria 20
  TMAO 83
Animal fats 30, 36, 46, 51, 54, 59, 64, 79, 83, 86, 145
Animal protein 48, 133, 134, 136, 137
Anti-aging x, 122, 126
Antibiotics 17, 91
  immune system viii, ix, x, 11, 19, 21, 23, 25, 27, 32, 39, 40, 42, 57, 85, 95, 118, 119, 121, 122, 129, 143, 158
Antibodies 33, 34, 37, 39, 41, 43, 55, 78, 85, 87
  Immune system viii, ix, x, 11, 19, 21, 23, 25, 27, 32, 39, 40, 42, 57, 85, 95, 118, 119, 121, 122, 129, 143, 158

Antigens 33, 42
Antioxidants xii, 14, 28, 38, 44, 49, 50, 56, 59, 61, 62, 63, 64, 74, 78, 86, 94, 95, 104, 116, 119, 125, 131, 144, 150, 151, 152, 153, 156, 158, 159, 160, 161, 162, 172, 178, 183
  best foods 1
  free radicals 14, 38, 45, 46, 56, 58, 65, 66, 68, 69, 74, 76, 81, 94, 95, 103, 106, 119, 122, 133, 134, 135, 140, 143, 145, 150, 156
Apoptosis 26, 126
Atherosclerosis 27, 44, 81
Autism 180
Avocado oil 38

B

Bacteria 7, 30, 39
  Microbiome 7, 30, 39
BCAAs (Branch Chain Amino Acids) xiv
  In supplements for athletes xiv, 135
  isoleucine, leucine, and valine 135
Beans 28, 37, 99, 134
Best diets viii
  Anti-inflammatory 7, 14, 19, 22, 37, 38, 42, 43, 45, 93, 119, 121, 122, 123, 125, 126, 127, 128, 144, 152, 156, 177
  biological age 42, 140, 147, 148, 165

Intermittent fasting viii, 42, 50
Reversing xi, 82, 83, 122, 133, 144
vegan 42, 43, 50, 60, 63, 101, 103, 135
Vegetarian 47, 48, 50, 60, 63, 64, 101, 116, 127
Bifidobacterium 23, 39, 130
Blood tests 34, 79, 98, 113
Blueberries 38, 44, 50, 62, 131, 156, 160, 162
Blue Zones xiv, 46, 47, 48, 49, 51, 86, 175
Boron 118, 120
Brain xi, 1, 5, 9, 10, 11, 12, 13, 14, 15, 16, 18, 19, 26, 40, 41, 54, 68, 69, 78, 89, 90, 99, 112, 115, 123, 124, 127, 141, 152, 153, 176, 179, 180
brain-gut connection 179
Broccoli 38
Bromelain 124, 125
Butyrate 19, 24, 25, 26, 27, 28, 176
  cancer 8, 19, 20, 22, 23, 25, 26, 28, 33, 35, 36, 37, 38, 42, 43, 45, 47, 48, 50, 53, 54, 56, 64, 65, 68, 69, 72, 74, 75, 76, 77, 79, 80, 81, 94, 95, 96, 102, 103, 104, 105, 106, 107, 109, 114, 119, 123, 125, 126, 128, 129, 135, 137, 145, 152, 168, 173, 178, 179
  diabetes Type 2 150
  IBS 7, 8, 13, 18, 22, 23, 25, 26, 33, 78
  inflammation ix, xii, 8, 14, 15, 18, 20, 23, 25, 27, 33, 35, 36, 37, 38, 39, 41, 42, 43, 45, 49, 51, 56, 68, 72, 74, 77, 78, 85, 86, 88, 90, 92, 93, 94, 106, 117, 118, 119, 120, 121, 122, 123, 125, 126, 127, 128, 130, 131, 137, 144, 145, 150, 152, 153, 154, 156, 157, 177, 179, 181, 182

C

Calcium 18, 82, 90, 92, 107, 108, 109, 110, 116, 117, 118, 120, 152, 156, 157, 160, 161, 162
Caloric restriction 61, 71, 81, 124
  AMPK 44, 50, 61, 71, 72, 128
  extended lifespan 72
  intermittent fasting 44, 50, 61, 68, 73, 135, 160
  weight loss 25, 31, 51, 64, 70, 72, 113
Cancer 8, 19, 20, 22, 23, 25, 26, 28, 33, 35, 36, 37, 38, 42, 43, 45, 47, 48, 50, 53, 54, 56, 64, 65, 68, 69, 72, 74, 75, 76, 77, 79, 80, 81, 94, 95, 96, 102, 103, 104, 105, 106, 107, 109, 114, 119, 123, 125, 126, 128, 129, 135, 137, 145, 152, 168, 173, 178, 179
Celiac disease 8, 33
Cholesterol 14, 19, 20, 22, 28, 36, 50, 64, 80, 82, 90, 107, 110, 111, 117, 120
Chromium 110, 111, 120, 156
Chronic diseases 6, 19, 47, 94, 137, 139, 149
Chronic inflammation ix, xii, 33, 36, 37, 38, 43, 51, 56, 77, 78, 88, 94, 120, 121, 122, 123, 137, 144, 145, 150, 152, 153, 154, 156, 181
  causes 7, 8, 20, 21, 32, 33, 35, 37, 65, 68, 73, 74, 75, 76, 77, 79, 80, 81, 95, 104, 107, 115, 118, 137
  Diets viii, ix, xi, xiii, xiv, xv, 19, 20, 29, 31, 32, 38, 39, 43, 44, 45, 46, 47, 48, 51, 54, 55, 56, 57, 59, 61, 63, 64, 66, 68, 80, 81, 82, 84, 85, 86, 89, 90, 95, 112, 120, 124, 134, 135, 136, 139, 140, 143, 145, 150, 151, 156, 159, 178, 182

leaky gut xiv, 8, 15, 32, 33, 34, 35, 37, 41, 42, 84, 122, 144, 145
Colon 4, 5, 7, 8, 18, 19, 20, 23, 24, 26, 27, 28, 36, 152, 179
Colon Cancer 172
 animal diets 19
CoQ10 90, 93, 94, 120

D

Dairy 8, 35, 43, 48, 50, 54, 63, 72, 76, 80, 83, 84, 86, 101, 111, 134, 135, 136, 152, 156, 179
Depression 8, 13, 16, 19, 23, 26, 73, 91, 92, 117, 120, 149, 158
 Anxiety 13, 91
 microbiome viii, ix, xiv, xv, 9, 10, 12, 14, 15, 17, 18, 27, 28, 29, 33, 36, 38, 39, 41, 43, 63, 64, 87, 105, 153, 154, 176
DHEA 90, 144
Dietary Guidelines 54, 79, 80
Diets viii, ix, xi, xiii, xiv, xv, 19, 20, 29, 31, 32, 38, 39, 43, 44, 45, 46, 47, 48, 51, 54, 55, 56, 57, 59, 61, 63, 64, 66, 68, 80, 81, 82, 84, 85, 86, 89, 90, 95, 112, 120, 124, 134, 135, 136, 139, 140, 143, 145, 150, 151, 156, 159, 178, 182
 anti-inflammatory 7, 14, 19, 22, 37, 38, 42, 43, 45, 93, 119, 121, 122, 123, 125, 126, 127, 128, 144, 152, 156, 177
 Blue Zones xiv, 46, 47, 48, 49, 51, 86, 175
 intermittent fasting 44, 50, 61, 68, 73, 135, 160
 Mediterranean 59, 172, 173
 Paleo 85, 86, 175
 plant-based xiv, 14, 19, 20, 42, 44, 46, 47, 48, 49, 50, 51, 54, 55, 57, 59, 60, 61, 63, 64, 82, 83, 84, 86, 87, 95, 124, 125, 134, 135, 136, 152, 159, 178, 181, 182
 rich in antioxidants 38, 44, 49, 50, 61, 63, 64, 74, 131, 144, 152, 153, 160
 vegan 42, 43, 50, 60, 63, 101, 103, 135
DNA x, 15, 38, 45, 51, 52, 53, 56, 58, 63, 65, 66, 68, 69, 74, 76, 85, 94, 98, 99, 106, 109, 116, 119, 124, 125, 128, 133, 134, 138, 139, 144, 145, 146, 148, 149, 165, 178, 179
DRESS-SS ix, 13, 49, 125, 135, 139, 147, 151, 154
 prescription viii, ix, 13, 40, 49, 53, 90, 94, 95, 113, 125, 135, 139, 147, 151, 154, 164

E

Eat right viii, 44
Eat Right i, xiii
Eggs 20, 43, 47, 48, 49, 50, 54, 60, 83, 86, 89, 98, 105, 106, 109, 110, 113, 134, 136, 159
 the enteric nervous system 16
 The enteric nervous system 16
Epigenome x, xi, 52, 125, 135, 138, 139, 146, 148, 149, 150, 151
 Gene expression 53
 Genome xi, xii, 52, 138, 148, 168

F

Fasting 42, 44, 50, 61, 67, 68, 73, 81, 135, 150, 160
Fast-keto diet 67, 68
Fats xiii, xiv, 4, 9, 14, 30, 31, 36, 37, 38, 43, 46, 49, 50, 51, 54, 55, 56, 59, 60, 61, 62, 64, 68, 72, 76, 77, 78, 79, 80, 81, 83, 86, 87, 89, 107, 116, 124, 136, 145, 150, 151, 162
Fermented foods 14, 24, 64
Flavonoids 38, 49, 53, 59, 62, 94, 125
Folic acid 39, 43, 54, 90, 91, 98, 99, 102, 115

deficiency 16, 35, 53, 54, 90, 91, 94, 95, 99, 100, 101, 102, 103, 104, 105, 107, 109, 111, 112, 113, 114, 115, 117, 118, 120, 135, 140, 177, 181, 182
  Methylation 45, 52, 53, 98, 125, 128, 148, 149, 165
Food sensitivity testing 42, 43
Foods rich in antioxidants 44
For pregnancy 100
Free radicals 14, 38, 45, 46, 56, 58, 65, 66, 68, 69, 74, 76, 81, 94, 95, 103, 106, 119, 122, 133, 134, 135, 140, 143, 145, 150, 156
Fruits 14, 29, 31, 38, 44, 50, 51, 53, 58, 59, 62, 63, 64, 76, 83, 84, 86, 87, 94, 95, 96, 98, 103, 104, 107, 108, 109, 111, 120, 126, 127, 128, 130, 131, 150, 153, 155, 156, 159, 162
Functional medicine 43, 94

G

Gallbladder 2, 3, 4, 7
Gene expression 53
  folate and B12 53
  rich in methyl groups 53
Gene Expression 141
Genes x, xii, 48, 52, 53, 66, 105, 119, 130, 135, 137, 138, 139, 140, 141, 148, 149, 150, 151
  Do We Have Aging Genes? 137
Genetic testing 94, 165
Genome xi, xii, 52, 138, 148, 168
  epigenome x, xi, 52, 125, 135, 138, 139, 146, 148, 149, 150, 151
GI map 41
Glucose 58, 65, 66, 75, 76, 111, 124
Gluten 8, 33, 35, 84, 86, 92
  Food allergies 92
  IBS 7, 8, 13, 18, 22, 23, 25, 26, 33, 78
Green tea 50, 53, 125, 131
Gut-brain connection 5, 9, 11, 12, 16, 40

Gut microbiome 10, 12, 14, 17, 63, 154
Gut permeability 35
  autoimmune diseases x, xiv, 15, 19, 33, 40, 42, 51, 121
  DNA methylation 45, 52, 53, 98, 125, 128, 149, 165
  food allergies 92
  leaky gut xiv, 8, 15, 32, 33, 34, 35, 37, 41, 42, 84, 122, 144, 145
  Occludin 33, 41
  Zonulin 33, 41, 42

H

H2 blockers 101
Hashimoto Thyroiditis 19
  autoimmune disease 34, 78, 101
  leaky gut xiv, 8, 15, 32, 33, 34, 35, 37, 41, 42, 84, 122, 144, 145
Health span 68, 133, 135, 140, 147, 151
Hormonal Dysregulation 141
Hypothalamus 140, 141, 142, 143

I

Intestine xiv, 2, 3, 4, 5, 7, 8, 11, 16, 24, 32, 34, 35, 89, 99, 102
intrinsic factor 99, 100, 101, 102
Iodine 90, 111, 112, 114, 182
iron 90, 92, 95, 103, 104, 108, 110, 112, 113, 114, 115, 116, 161, 162

J

Junk foods 36, 61
  heart disease xi, xiv, 36, 37, 42, 45, 47, 48, 61, 63, 64, 77, 80, 82, 83, 84, 94, 96, 99, 103, 138, 149, 152
  obesity xiii, xiv, 18, 21, 26, 32, 36, 37, 38, 43, 45, 55, 58, 59, 61, 62, 63, 64, 65, 69, 75, 77, 79, 80, 84, 136, 172, 173

K

ketoacidosis 73, 74
Ketosis 67, 68, 73

L

Lactobacillus plantarum PS128 91
  Anxiety and depression 13
  Autism 13, 79, 81, 89, 91, 92, 180
  Food allergies 92
  food sensitivities xiv, xv, 33, 34, 38, 41, 42, 43, 77, 78, 79, 87
  leaky gut xiv, 8, 15, 32, 33, 34, 35, 37, 41, 42, 84, 122, 144, 145
  Occludin 33, 41
  Parkinson's Disease 13, 91
  tests for 93
  Zonulin 33, 34, 92
Leaky Gut 34, 35, 40
Lectins 37, 84, 85, 86
Legumes 21, 47, 49, 84, 85, 86, 87, 116
Life expectancy 48, 80
Lifespan and health span 68, 135, 140
Liver 2, 3, 4, 7, 8, 35, 58, 61, 67, 72, 73, 75, 76, 105, 108, 109, 115, 124

M

Magnesium 38, 53, 90, 91, 92, 94, 108, 110, 113, 116, 117, 118, 157, 158, 161, 162, 177
  Zinc 53, 90, 91, 93, 94, 107, 110, 113, 118, 119, 120, 145, 158, 162
Metformin 17, 75, 102
Methionine xiv, 49, 86, 133, 134, 135
  Lifespan ix, xiv, 9, 36, 46, 49, 52, 68, 72, 124, 131, 134, 135, 136, 138, 140, 146, 147, 151
Methylation 45, 52, 53, 98, 125, 128, 148, 149, 165
Methyl donors 53
Microbiome viii, ix, xiv, xv, 9, 10, 12, 14, 15, 17, 18, 27, 28, 29, 33, 36, 38, 39, 41, 43, 63, 64, 87, 105, 153, 154, 176
  as Dietary Supplements 21
  As Oncobiotics 39, 40
  As Psychobiotic 39, 40
  Best Foods for 38
  Foods iii, vii, xii, xiii, xiv, 1, 8, 11, 14, 15, 17, 18, 19, 20, 21, 22, 24, 25, 26, 27, 28, 30, 31, 32, 33, 34, 35, 36, 37, 38, 39, 40, 41, 42, 43, 44, 45, 46, 47, 49, 50, 51, 52, 53, 54, 55, 59, 60, 61, 62, 64, 72, 76, 77, 78, 80, 81, 84, 85, 86, 87, 88, 92, 95, 98, 99, 101, 104, 107, 109, 110, 111, 112, 113, 114, 116, 118, 120, 125, 130, 131, 132, 134, 135, 136, 144, 150, 151, 152, 155, 172
  omega-3 38, 39, 43, 50, 63, 80, 86, 90, 93, 94, 123, 156, 157, 158, 161
  pharmabiotics 40
  Prebiotics 14, 18, 19, 27, 29, 39, 89
  probiotics 5, 14, 16, 17, 18, 20, 21, 23, 24, 29, 39, 40, 42, 64, 89, 91, 92, 153, 154, 160, 161, 176, 177
  Synbiotics 40
Minerals xv, 9, 29, 45, 54, 56, 59, 62, 78, 88, 89, 90, 91, 92, 93, 94, 108, 109, 110, 112, 115, 118, 120, 131, 151, 156, 157, 159, 160, 161, 177
  iodine 90, 109, 111, 112, 113, 114, 182
  Iron 90, 92, 95, 103, 104, 108, 110, 112, 113, 114, 115, 116, 161, 162
Mitochondrial theory 134
MSM 121, 122, 123, 181
Mycotoxins 14, 17, 43, 77, 78, 79, 80, 81, 87, 88, 92, 154
  Testing 51, 164, 165

N

NAC 93, 123
NAD+ and NMN 123
Neurotransmitters 148
Nutrients 54, 180, 181
   deficiencies ix, 16, 18, 46, 54, 55, 83, 87, 88, 89, 90, 94, 95, 105, 111, 112, 113, 115, 116, 118, 119, 120, 121, 154

O

Obesity xiii, xiv, 13, 18, 21, 26, 32, 36, 37, 38, 43, 45, 55, 58, 59, 61, 62, 63, 64, 65, 69, 75, 77, 79, 80, 84, 136, 167, 172, 173, 180
Omega-3 121, 123, 161
Osteoporosis 142
Oxidative stress 74
Ozempic 31, 32, 70, 178
   GLP-1 70

P

Pancreas 3, 4
Parkinson's disease 26, 81, 89
plant-based foods 14, 19, 46, 47, 54, 59, 95, 135
polyphenols 38, 53, 56, 63, 94, 124, 130, 150, 160
Prebiotic foods 27
Prebiotics 14, 18, 19, 27, 29, 39, 89
Prevotella species 19
Probiotics 14, 16, 17, 18, 20, 21, 39, 89, 180

Q

Quercetin 49, 53, 59, 126, 127, 128, 129
   Foods rich in Quercetin 127
   In periodontal disease 129
   periodontitis 126, 127, 128, 129
   senolytic x, 126, 127, 129

R

Recipes xv, 64
Rectum 5, 6, 7
References 167
Resources ix, xv, 113
resveratrol x, 126, 129, 177
Reversing Aging viii, 32, 151, 154

S

Salmon 38, 39, 43, 49, 50, 105, 109, 117, 118, 135, 159, 160, 162, 177
Saturated fats xiii, xiv, 14, 31, 37, 38, 46, 49, 50, 54, 55, 56, 59, 60, 61, 72, 76, 77, 80, 86, 124, 136, 150
Selenium 90, 94, 107, 108, 109, 157, 158, 159, 182
Serotonin 12, 16, 91, 117, 162
SIBO 16
Skin aging 131, 142, 143, 144
Sleep 11, 27, 49, 50, 51, 53, 69, 92, 117, 118, 122, 141, 150, 162
Smoothies xv, 50, 58, 59, 62, 63, 64, 123, 150, 156, 159
Stem cells 121, 143, 145, 151, 153
Stomach vii, 2, 3, 7, 8, 9, 10, 11, 20, 24, 30, 41, 70, 99, 101, 102, 109, 114, 115, 121
Stomach acid 24, 101, 102
Stress ix, 11, 74, 151, 178
Sugar 3, 4, 8, 14, 19, 26, 27, 28, 35, 43, 44, 45, 46, 47, 51, 54, 57, 58, 59, 61, 62, 63, 65, 66, 67, 68, 69, 70, 75, 76, 80, 85, 89, 110, 117, 136, 150, 157, 158, 163
Supplements viii, ix, xiv, xv, 20, 22, 24, 25, 26, 29, 31, 40, 45, 53, 84, 88, 90, 93, 95, 96, 98, 99, 100, 102, 104, 109, 110, 113, 114, 118, 120, 121, 124, 131, 135, 144, 153, 154, 176, 177, 181

T

Testing xv, 34, 42, 43, 87, 88, 93, 94, 108, 145, 164, 165
TMAO (trimethylamine-N-oxide) 20
Turmeric 50, 53, 168
Type 2 diabetes 21, 47, 52, 55, 66, 69, 81, 102

V

Vagus nerve 9, 10, 12, 16
Vegan diet 42, 43, 50, 63, 101, 103, 135
Vegetables 14, 31, 38, 39, 49, 50, 51, 53, 54, 59, 61, 62, 63, 64, 76, 83, 84, 86, 94, 95, 96, 98, 99, 104, 106, 107, 108, 109, 111, 117, 120, 126, 127, 128, 130, 131, 135, 150, 153, 155, 156, 159, 170
Vegetarian diet 48, 50, 60, 63, 64
Vitamin A 180
Vitamin B complex 43
Vitamin C 50, 63, 90, 91, 92, 93, 94, 95, 103, 104, 111, 116, 119
Vitamin D 93, 98, 105, 142, 143, 171, 182
Vitamin E 171
Vitamin K 107, 108
Vitamins 177

W

Wellness lifestyle 51, 80, 125, 139
Wrinkles 21, 95, 103, 106, 119, 122, 142, 143, 163

Y

Yamanaka factors 133
Yogurt 160, 161

Z

Zinc 53, 90, 91, 93, 94, 107, 110, 113, 118, 119, 120, 145, 158, 162

www.ingramcontent.com/pod-product-compliance
Lightning Source LLC
LaVergne TN
LVHW061545070526
838199LV00077B/6902